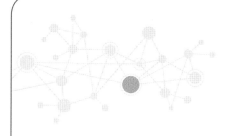

FYI™
For Learning Agility
A Must-Have Resource for High Potential Development

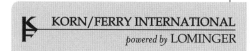

Swisher, Hallenbeck, Orr, Eichinger, Lombardo & Capretta

FYI™ FOR LEARNING AGILITY
2nd Edition

ISBN 978-1-933578-49-1

Item number 82199

FYI™ for Learning Agility Printings:
version 10.1a—01/10

FYI™ for Learning Agility 2nd edition
version 13.1a—04/13

Printed in the United States

Table of Contents

Introduction

A fundamental shift has taken place in the world of work. Permanent forces of change are taking hold in the form of globalization, technological shifts, and economic and political uncertainty. Everything's faster, more interconnected, complex, and ambiguous than ever before. As a result, the era of job stability and predictability is now a thing of the past.

The only way to survive, let alone thrive, in the face of such overwhelming change is to adapt at the same pace of the change, if not even faster. This means being able to develop new skills in the blink of an eye, to face unfamiliar challenges without a "playbook" to guide you, to find an answer when the problem itself isn't clear. In short, it means you have to become adept at knowing what to do when you don't know what to do.

But how do you do that? The secret is something called *Learning Agility*. Individuals who excel at Learning Agility have mastered the ability to effectively learn from their experiences. They embrace what happens to them, both good and bad, and look for the key takeaways and lessons learned. And they don't stop there. They seek ways to actively apply those lessons, especially to new and difficult challenges that they face.

Learning Agility is a well-defined set of behaviors that has been studied for several decades. While skill at Learning Agility does vary, it is an ability that can be developed, primarily through seeking and gaining from experiences that build breadth and adaptability. This book breaks down the specific elements of Learning Agility and provides a practical, actionable approach to developing what has now become one of the must-have skills for workplace success.

WHO IS THIS BOOK FOR?
This book was designed for any motivated person seeking to develop skills that lead to increased Learning Agility. The suggestions provided are aimed at gaining insight and strength in specific areas where Learning Agility needs to be developed. It does not matter what level of the organization you are a part of or what type of industry or function you are in. If you perceive that Learning Agility is important to your current and future success and you are committed to developing, this book is for you. In addition to individual learners, the content will also help anyone who is serving as a manager, mentor, or feedback giver.

Timing is important. Do make certain that you are ready to develop. The earliest and most critical stages in the development process are the awareness and acceptance of the need to develop. If you are in denial, rationalizing, confused, or being defensive about having needs, this book will not help.

Awareness and acceptance aren't enough though. You also need to be motivated. Individuals who accept that they have a need to increase their Learning Agility but do not have the motivation, drive, urgency, or energy to do anything about it will also not be helped by what's in this book.

So, this book is intended for people who believe they have a need and want to do something about it. If this describes you, there are hundreds of tips in this book that will help you develop skills that lead to increased Learning Agility.

THE STRUCTURE OF THIS BOOK:
Each of the 27 chapters addresses one of the dimensions of Learning Agility and includes the following sections:

1. **Map** – At the beginning of each dimension chapter, the map explains key elements of the dimension and their importance.

2. **Quotations** – Quotations are provided at the beginning and end of each dimension chapter for the purpose of inspiration and reflection.

3. **Definition** – What Skilled, Less Skilled, and Overuse look like for this dimension of Learning Agility.

4. **Some Possible Causes of Lower Skill** – We list numerous reasons why you might have this need. Use these to specify what your need looks like exactly.

5. **Developmental Difficulty** – Each dimension is classified as Easier ◢ or Moderate ◢ or Harder ◢ to develop. This will help you set your expectations regarding the scope and speed of your development.

6. **Did You Know ?/ Does It Best** ★ Each dimension is highlighted with research-related insights or a brief portrait of someone who serves as a prime example of skilled behavior.

7. **Tips to Increase Skill** – Research- and experience-based suggestions for actions that you can take to increase effectiveness in each dimension. Choose a few to include in your development plan. Also consult the Resources to Learn More for more tips and deeper understanding.

   Look for this symbol for tips on how to avoid ***overusing*** your skill in each dimension.

8. **Assignments to Practice Skill** – Ideas for ways to pursue developmental opportunities in the dimension both on and off the job.

9. **Take Time to Reflect** – Each chapter closes with a series of thought-provoking questions to inspire further reflection on the dimension and raise your level of self-awareness.

HOW DO I USE THIS BOOK?

There are several practices and approaches we find useful for getting the most out of this book:

Determine the need. From regular feedback or use of the Learning Agility Architect™ Sort Cards, Quick Score Questionnaire, or Choices™ online assessment, try to determine your current level of Learning Agility and which areas you could benefit from working on. Sometimes even excellent feedback can identify the wrong need. Even if everyone agrees that you have problems managing conflict, the question is "Why?" Maybe the real problem is due to your not being open to others' opinions or not being able to read people's reactions. So if none or only a few of the tips for your identified need seem to make sense, check other likely dimensions to see if the need is more likely one of those.

Get the lay of the land. Read the map for the dimension at the start of each chapter. The map describes the general case of the behavior, how it operates, and why it's important. The map sets context and helps clarify what the dimension is all about.

Specify the need. Read the Less Skilled definition for the dimension. Which bullet points describe your particular situation best? Look to the Skilled definition. How do you want to act when you have developed in this dimension? This is the before and after picture. Also consider the potential for Overuse.

3

Ask "Why?" Check the Possible Causes that might apply. Many developmental efforts have floundered because the plan attacked the wrong problem. Causes get to "why" you may have a need in this dimension. Write down your specific need—what it looks like, what causes it, who it plays out with, and in what situations.

Conduct a reality check. Take note of the Developmental Difficulty level of the dimension. Some weaknesses are tougher to fix than others. Knowing the relative difficulty of working on a need will help set you up for success.

Identify the fixes. Look at the Tips to Increase Skill and pick the specific ones that apply. Each topic is written against a specific manifestation of being less skilled at the dimension. It is unlikely that all of the topics or remedies will apply to any person. Pick a few that apply. Start small. Think back to the causes you checked and the "why it's important" noted from the map.

Seek out more knowledge. Look at the list of recommended Resources to Learn More. They might also be helpful to deepen your understanding on your needs and to help put together the action plan. *Complete Web addresses appear in the Resources to Learn More – Web Addresses appendix.*

Get ready. Get set… Lay out a plan and a schedule. The plan should include at least three items you will work on immediately. Use the development plan in the back of this book. Measure the number of times you do this or don't do that and record these efforts so you can track improvement. Set a specific time frame of no more than a month to try these items repeatedly. If the time frame is longer or indefinite, you will be less likely to do anything. Start today.

Begin the journey. Make it a journey of challenge. It's simply the most effective way to learn. In particular, put these practices to work for maximum learning gain:

Go against your natural grain. We call these GAG (Going Against your natural Grain). GAG because, while it's great for your development, it's uncomfortable. If you're ambitious or if you seek a different kind of job, you'll have to work on your downsides more vigorously. Few succeed in a different job by simply repeating past successful behavior. This is a strong lesson from career research. You'll have to stretch in uncomfortable areas. For example, whether you gravitate toward team building or not, you can learn the behaviors of excellent team builders. You might even come to enjoy it. It's important not to confuse what you like to do with what's necessary to do.

Test the unknown. Many Learning Agility dimensions you might be low on reflect lack of experience that we call an untested area. Maybe you don't deal with change well but have never led a change effort. Pick something small that needs doing and give it a try using the tips from the dimensions that are a part of Change Agility.

Seek further feedback. Little happens without feedback tied to a goal. Get a developmental partner, get feedback a year from now on the Choices™ online assessment, ask for a Learning From Experience™ interview, poll people you work with about what you should keep doing, keep doing with slight modifications, stop doing, and start doing.

Finally, remember that Learning Agility is forged by experience. Experiences are needed to provide the seeds for learning and even more experiences are needed to provide opportunities to apply and refine those learnings. So be patient and stay committed to continually embracing, reflecting on, and applying whatever can be gleaned from the many experiences that await you.

About the Authors

VICTORIA V. SWISHER

Vicki Swisher is Senior Director of Intellectual Property Development for Korn/Ferry International. She is author of *Becoming an Agile Leader: Know What to Do…When You Don't Know What to Do* and co-author of *FYI™ for Teams* 2nd Edition and *FYI™ for Insight: The 21 Leadership Characteristics for Success and the 5 That Get You Fired*. Vicki has extensive experience in the areas of leadership development and talent management. She has written several articles and both teaches and frequently speaks on the topics of Learning Agility and leadership development at premier talent management events around the world. Prior to Korn/Ferry, Vicki held internal consulting and leadership positions with top companies in the financial services and hospitality sectors.

GEORGE S. HALLENBECK JR.

George Hallenbeck is Vice President of Intellectual Property Development at Korn/Ferry International. He is co-author of several books, including *Selecting an Agile Leader: Find Future-Ready Talent Today, Interviewing Right: How Science Can Sharpen Your Interviewing Accuracy, FYI™ for Insight: The 21 Leadership Characteristics for Success and the 5 That Get You Fired*, and *The CIO Edge: Seven Leadership Skills You Need to Drive Results*. George is a frequent speaker on emerging trends and critical issues in talent and has authored or co-authored numerous white papers and scientific articles on Learning Agility. He has extensive experience consulting with companies in Asia, including an extended assignment in Singapore.

J. EVELYN ORR

Evelyn Orr is Director of Intellectual Property Development at Korn/Ferry International. She is author of *Becoming an Agile Leader: A Guide to Learning From Your Experiences* and co-author of several publications, including the books *Selecting an Agile Leader: Find Future-Ready Talent Today, FYI™ for Insight: The 21 Leadership Characteristics for Success and the 5 That Get You Fired*, and *Paths to Improvement: Navigating Your Way to Success*. With over a decade of experience in leadership development and talent management, Evelyn is highly skilled at assessing and developing leaders' Learning Agility. Prior to Korn/Ferry, Evelyn held leadership positions in a large retail organization and has consulted with multiple Fortune 500 companies from a variety of industries.

ROBERT W. EICHINGER

Bob Eichinger is co-founder and former CEO of Lominger International. Along with Mike Lombardo, Bob is the creator and seminal thought leader of the Learning Agility concept. In addition to the groundbreaking research and comprehensive application tools for Learning Agility, Bob co-created the Leadership Architect® suite of management, executive, and organizational development tools. During his 40+ year career, he has worked inside companies such as PepsiCo and Pillsbury, and as a consultant in multiple Fortune 500 companies. Bob continues to lecture extensively around the world on the topic of leader development. Of his many books and publications, two of his most notable include *The Leadership Machine* and the million-selling *FYI™ For Your Improvement*, both co-written with fellow Lominger founder Mike Lombardo.

MICHAEL M. LOMBARDO

Mike Lombardo is co-founder of Lominger International, during which time he and Bob Eichinger created the research-based Learning Agility concept. Along with his foundational contributions to both the thought leadership and application of Learning Agility, Mike is co-creator of The Leadership Architect®, a comprehensive suite of leadership development tools that has been adding value to organizations globally for almost 25 years. With Bob Eichinger, Mike has authored over 40 products, including *The Leadership Machine, FYI™ For Your Improvement,* and the Learning Agility Architect™ (formerly Choices Architect®) solution. Mike is co-author of *The Lessons of Experience* that detailed which learnings from experience lead to executive success. He also co-authored the research on executive derailment revealing how personal flaws and overdone strengths can lead to career trouble.

CARA C. CAPRETTA

Cara Capretta is former President and Chief Operating Officer of Lominger International and co-author of several Lominger publications, including *FYI™ for Teams* 2nd Edition and The Interview Architect®. Cara has over 20 years of practical experience working with leaders, teams, and organizations. In her current role as Vice President – Human Capital Management (HCM) Transformation Practice at Oracle, Cara continues to use her deep expertise in Learning Agility to help organizations best identify and develop their high potential talent.

Fundamentals of Learning Agility

*When the winds of change rage, some build shelters
while others build windmills.*

A Chinese Proverb

"So what makes you think Viktor is a high potential?"

"Well, he is an outstanding performer. He blew away the top line numbers last year and was still able to keep costs down. He's the expert we rely on. He always does what I ask him to do. He gets along with everyone at the company. He's a great mentor. He'd be tough to replace, that's for sure!"

And...

"Viktor consistently volunteers to work overtime and comes in on weekends if I need him. He always has a smile on his face. In fact, one time last year when I was in the hospital and missed a week of work, Viktor managed the department seamlessly. I can depend on him."

Such conversations occur every year during talent review meetings in organizations around the world. Managers strongly perceive some of their employees to be high potentials and seek to groom them for senior-level executive positions. In their eyes, these employees have "the right stuff." But do they really? Are we sure? How do we know? And if they really are high potentials, how should we develop them so they can be ready for future promotions?

The development of a company's future leaders is widely recognized as a top business priority in most organizations today (Blanchard, 2007; Dychtwald, Erickson, & Morison, 2006). Unfortunately, many companies appear to do a poor job at identifying which employees truly are high potentials. According to several recent studies, only about one-half of companies report having a high potential identification program (Howard, 2009; Slan-Jerusalim & Hausdorf, 2007; Wells, 2003). And those companies which do have programs frequently select individuals based on factors not necessarily related to potential, such as personal experience with the person, performance review ratings, and past performance results (Slan-Jerusalim & Hausdorf, 2007; Pepermans, Vloeberghs, & Perkisas, 2003). Even when companies do select the right employees, their subsequent development often is unsystematic and ineffective.

8

Many corporate executives candidly admit that they are dissatisfied with their company's initiatives for developing leaders (Charan, 2005). The issue is *not* that companies don't develop people. Development happens in all companies. Rather, the real issue is that development is not planful or systematic. Many companies don't understand how development happens. They don't know when to develop which competencies in what situations. Worse yet, they identify the wrong people for development. That is not to say that companies shouldn't view all of their employees as important. Obviously, they are. However, some employees have much more potential for future leadership positions than others. In particular, organizations should focus on differentiated leadership development programs to build skills for those high potentials.

The proper assessment, identification, and development of high potentials represents one of the key components of best-in-class leadership development programs (Hewitt Associates, 2005). In this chapter, we review what makes an employee a high potential or so-called "hipo." We make an important distinction between a high potential, a high professional, and a high performer. We introduce the term *Learning Agility* as a key indicator of leadership potential and articulate its historical background. The Choices™ assessment is presented as a psychometrically validated instrument of the concept and relevant empirical findings are highlighted. Finally, we discuss how Learning Agility can be used to develop the next generation of leaders in the workforce.

DISTINGUISHING BETWEEN HIGH POTENTIALS, HIGH PROFESSIONALS, AND HIGH PERFORMERS

High potentials are people with some specific characteristics. Sure, they perform their jobs exceedingly well. They are competent. They are dependable and reliable. They are motivated. They willingly volunteer to be on nearly any task force or assignment that must be done. They go the extra mile. However, more importantly, they are agile learners—they like experimenting, trying new things. They are highly curious. Research suggests the following characteristics are common among high potential employees:

- Easily learn new tasks and functions
- Enjoy and deal well with ambiguity and complexity
- Don't accept the status quo
- Are impatient
- Like to try new things, different approaches
- Tend to push the envelope
- Are willing to take the heat when things fail

Such employees are excellent candidates for senior general management and leadership positions.

In contrast, *high professionals* are functional or technical experts in a defined area or function. They have a proven track record of superior performance year after year. The following characteristics are common among high professionals:

- Are passionate about what they do
- Love their role in the organization and the contributions they make
- Likely possess a depth of organizational knowledge
- Are viewed as trusted resources within the organization
- Are widely recognized outside the company for their knowledge and expertise
- Tend to be excellent at mentoring and developing people
- Frequently do not aspire to broader management roles

Both high potentials and high professionals are critical to an organization's future success. Both can be difficult to replace. Obviously, both are needed. However, their organizational contributions—current and future—are quite different.

In addition, we need to understand that there is a clear difference between *high performers* and high potentials. Not all high performers are high potentials. Research suggests that only about 30% of high performers can be classified as high potentials (Corporate Leadership Council, 2005). Also worth noting is that not all high potentials are high performers, but the percentage is much, much higher. The same study found that about 93% of high potentials perform at a high level.

LEARNING AGILITY: A PRIMARY INDICATOR OF HIGH POTENTIAL

In 2000, Michael Lombardo and Robert Eichinger published an article entitled "High Potentials as High Learners." It highlighted the concept of Learning Agility and presented their findings on the relationship between Learning Agility and leadership potential. The authors theorized that potential cannot be fully detected from what an individual already demonstrates on the job. Rather, it requires that the individual do something new or different. In the view of Lombardo and Eichinger, potential involves learning new skills to perform in new, very often first-time, situations. They speculated that people differ in their aptitude to learn from their experiences. It is this capability to learn from experience which differentiates high potentials from others (McCall, Lombardo, & Morrison, 1988).

The implication is that organizations should assess individuals' Learning Agility to identify truly high potentials for future leadership positions. This approach differed from most traditional practices at that time. Previously, most companies developed and promoted their high performers without realizing that current performance in one situation does not guarantee high performance in a different one. As mentioned, it has been observed that less than 30% of an organization's high performers have the *potential* to rise to and succeed in broader senior-level, critical positions. Consequently, organizations would be wise to strengthen their high potential assessment by adding Learning Agility to an individual's success profile. According to Lombardo and Eichinger, organizations need to measure "the willingness and ability to learn new competencies in order to perform under first-time, tough, or different conditions" (2000, p. 323).

Many different researchers have contributed to the evolution of Learning Agility as an important predictor of high potential identification. The longitudinal studies conducted at AT&T observed that people who had been assessed as having low potential frequently were more successful than expected if they had developmental opportunities (see Howard & Bray, 1988, Bray, Campbell, & Grant, 1974). Sternberg and his colleagues emphasized "practical intelligence" as a critical part of overall intelligence (Sternberg, 1984, 1997; Sternberg, Wagner, Williams, & Horvath, 1995). Such characteristics as being street smart, interpersonally savvy, and possessing common sense were important in "practical intelligence" or "learning intelligence." These authors found that learning intelligence (i.e., Learning Agility) was much more predictive of individual success than basic IQ.

Research and application of Learning Agility is not limited to certain industries or types of organizations. For example, the United States military has shown a particular interest in identifying and developing learning agile leaders. The military's mission in both conflict and peacekeeping activities has evolved considerably in recent years. Today, military personnel are required to play multiple roles, often during the course of a single day. Adaptability and agile learning are essential to navigate the situations soldiers face on a continuous basis. The difference in these cases, literally, could be life or death. Many of the findings from the military's research can be applied to the development of Learning Agility in other settings. Wong (2004) focused on the environmental drivers that promote the development of adaptive behaviors and identified the key elements of complexity, unpredictability, and ambiguity. Officers who responded constructively to these elements demonstrated higher levels of independence, initiative, innovation, and confidence. Gehler (2005) concluded that agile leaders need to be supported by agile institutions. Specifically,

Gehler suggested that training efforts need to be accelerated, dynamic, and experience-based to support the development of agile capabilities. Mueller-Hanson, White, Dorsey, and Pulakos (2005) recommended early and frequent exposure to training experiences that call for adaptive responses. They indicated soldiers should have numerous and diverse opportunities to apply the lessons learned, receive feedback, and then apply again.

In general, the formulation of the concept of Learning Agility is rooted largely in two streams of research. Both groups of research studies were conducted at the Center for Creative Leadership (CCL). One series of studies, referred to as "The Lessons of Experience," examined which leadership competencies were most important for success in organizational promotions. The other series of studies investigated reasons why executives derail. We review both research streams in the next section of this chapter.

THE LESSONS OF EXPERIENCE

By the early 1980s, researchers gradually recognized that it was not possible to provide a comprehensive summary of predisposing characteristics of effective leadership. Leadership seemed to be a product of growing up and gaining managerial experience. However, researchers continued to have a limited knowledge of how experience actually develops managers. Not all experiences appeared to be created equal. The question remained: "What experiences have the most developmental impact?" And, "Who will benefit most from such experiences?" Without understanding how people learn and grow from their experiences, organizations cannot fully take advantage of work-related assignments and job tasks as developmental opportunities.

CCL conducted a series of studies to understand how executives learn from their work experiences. Corporate executives were interviewed and asked to describe key events in their careers that caused the most learning. The following two questions were probed: (1) What specifically happened on the job, and (2) What did they learn from the event. Researchers interviewed 191 executives from six major corporations. Descriptions of the 616 events and 1,547 corresponding lessons were tabulated. The analyses and results are summarized in the book aptly titled *The Lessons of Experience* (McCall et al., 1988). Two findings had a lasting impact on the practice of leadership development. First, the rule of 70:20:10 was coined. It was discovered that approximately 70% of leadership development occurs primarily from job assignments, 20% from people, and only a small portion (roughly 10%) from traditional classroom education. Subsequently, this rule has been supported by other studies (see McCall & Hollenbeck, 2002).

The second important finding—one that is the most relevant here—is that people significantly differ as learners from experience. Some individuals learn more content than others. Learning and development requires that individuals move away from their comfort zone, habits, and routines. The researchers observed that the most developmental experiences are challenging, stretching, and difficult. The best learning experiences are emotional, require us to take risks, and tend to have real life consequences (Lombardo & Eichinger, 2011). The journey tends to be unpleasant. Learners have to be resilient and non-defensive. Individuals have to possess a strong need for growth. Overall, this research reveals that the willingness and ability to learn from experience separates high potentials from others. The importance of learning from experience for successful executives has been echoed by many other leadership researchers (e.g., Bennis & Thomas, 2002).

EXECUTIVE DERAILMENT
A second stream of research that framed the development of Learning Agility was conducted at CCL over two decades ago (Lombardo & Eichinger, 1989; Lombardo, Ruderman, & McCauley, 1988; McCall & Lombardo, 1983; Morrison, White, & Van Velsor, 1987, rev. 1992; Van Velsor & Leslie, 1995). These studies compared successful versus derailed executives. Derailed executives were defined as those individuals who were identified as high potentials, promoted, often promoted again, only to ultimately fail. This research produced consistent findings across time, hierarchical levels, national culture, gender, and organizations.

Overall, the authors found that *both* successful and derailed executives were: (a) very bright, (b) had been identified as high potentials *early* in their career, (c) possessed outstanding records of achievement, and (d) were ambitious and willing to sacrifice. Both groups of executives also possessed very few personal flaws. However, one derailment factor was observed repeatedly. The authors found that derailed executives were unable or unwilling to change or adapt. They relied too much on a narrow set of work skills. The derailed leaders generally had a series of prior successes but typically in very similar organizational situations. On the other hand, successful executives usually had a diverse set of experiences in a variety of settings. For most of the leaders who had derailed, their comparative technical superiority was a source of success at lower levels of leadership. However, when they ascended to the higher levels, this strength became a weakness, leading to overconfidence and arrogance. Successful and derailed executives also differed in the way they managed hardship and mistakes. Those executives who were successful overwhelmingly handled failure with poise and grace. They admitted mistakes, accepted responsibility, and then acted to correct the problems. In contrast, leaders who derailed tended to be defensive about their failure, attempting to keep it under cover while they fixed it, or they tended to blame others. Their unwillingness and/or inability to learn from experience appeared to be the major reason why they derailed.

The popular literature reveals similar stories of failed leaders. In his book, *Why Smart Executives Fail*, Sydney Finkelstein (2003) focused on a specialized subset of derailed executives—CEOs. He summarized the findings in terms of "the seven habits of spectacularly unsuccessful people" (p. 238). A few of the habits are directly related to Learning Agility, such as having all the answers and relying on what worked for them in the past. Goldsmith and Reiter (2007) advised executives "what got you here won't get you there." To continue down the path of success, successful leaders need to change, adapt, grow, and develop.

LEARNING AGILITY: WHAT IS IT? HOW DO WE DEFINE IT?

Learning Agility can be defined as *the ability and willingness to learn from experience, and subsequently apply that learning to perform successfully under new or first-time conditions*. Highly learning agile individuals learn the right lessons from experience and apply those learnings to new situations (Lombardo & Eichinger, 2000). Learning Agility is an important element of potential. Our research indicates that those individuals with greater Learning Agility are significantly more successful *after* they are promoted than others.

Learning Agility is different from intelligence or simply "being smart" (Eichinger & Lombardo, 2004; Sternberg et al., 1995). An individual's intelligence refers to his/her general mental capability and encompasses many related abilities, such as the capacity to reason, plan, solve problems, and think abstractly. Intelligence often is measured in terms of IQ (Intelligence Quotient). Being smart clearly does not guarantee managerial success (Hogan & Kaiser, 2005). Some may adopt a narrow definition of Learning Agility, such as viewing it as a specific cognitive ability (e.g., DeRue, Ashford, & Myers, 2012). However, learning from experience is full of socially contextual elements (De Meuse, Dai, Swisher, Eichinger, & Lombardo, 2012). Adversity or "hard knocks" is inevitable in this type of learning (Snell, 1992). Motivation and managing emotion are, therefore, some of the defining characteristics of Learning Agility (Arun, Coyle, & Hauenstein, 2012; Carette & Anseel, 2012; Hezlett & Kuncel, 2012).

The concept that leaders need to be learning agile has been broadly recognized and accepted in the management field (see Kaiser, 2008; Kaiser, Lindberg, & Craig, 2007; Spreitzer, McCall, & Mahoney, 1997). People who are highly agile continuously seek out new challenges, actively seek feedback from others to grow and develop, tend to self-reflect, and evaluate their experiences and draw practical conclusions. Although intelligence impacts the ability to learn from a traditional perspective, individuals who are learning agile tend to be active, continuous learners throughout their lifetime. Table 1 highlights the differences between traditional learners and active learners.

TABLE 1: CHARACTERISTICS OF TRADITIONAL AND ACTIVE LEARNERS

TRADITIONAL LEARNERS	ACTIVE LEARNERS
· High intellect	· Street smarts
· High grades, GPA, class rank	· High initiative and motivation
· Score well on tests (e.g., ACT, GRE)	· Intellectually flexible
· High functional/technical skills	· High conceptual complexity
· High verbal and analytical skills	· Very broad thinkers
· Linear problem solver	· Highly curious – why and how
· May or may not be self-aware	· High self-awareness

Leadership development entails a sequence of managerial transitions (Freedman, 1998). Transition often is challenging—and developmental—due to the fact that individuals are faced with novel situations rendering existing routines and leadership behaviors inadequate. It requires the flexibility to learn new ways of coping with unforeseen problems and opportunities (McCauley, Ruderman, Ohlott, & Morrow, 1994; De Meuse, Dai, & Hallenbeck, 2010). Individuals who can't let go of old patterns of behavior or who do not recognize the nuances in different situations tend to fail. To summarize McCall et al. (1988) and the book *The Lessons of Experience*:

....

The glaring difference between successful people
and those whose careers falter
...is their ability to wrest meaning from experience.

....

Learning Agility is widely posited as a multidimensional concept. Based on many years of research, Korn/Ferry International developed a model of Learning Agility that consists of the following five factors: Self-Awareness, Mental Agility, People Agility, Change Agility, and Results Agility. Each factor consists of five to six dimensions. Subsequent chapters will articulate the factors and dimensions in detail. Figure 1 depicts the five-factor model of Learning Agility.

Figure 1: Five Factors of Learning Agility

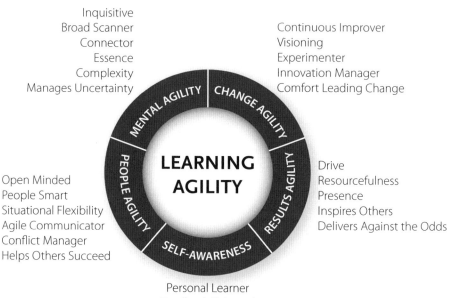

Inquisitive
Broad Scanner
Connector
Essence
Complexity
Manages Uncertainty

Continuous Improver
Visioning
Experimenter
Innovation Manager
Comfort Leading Change

Open Minded
People Smart
Situational Flexibility
Agile Communicator
Conflict Manager
Helps Others Succeed

Drive
Resourcefulness
Presence
Inspires Others
Delivers Against the Odds

Personal Learner
Feedback Oriented
Reflective
Emotion Management
Self-Knowledge

Multi-Rater Assessment of Learning Agility

CHOICES™

Choices™ is a multi-rater assessment of Learning Agility. The instrument consists of 81 items assessing 27 dimensions and five factors of Learning Agility. A significant feature of the instrument is that the items describe observable behaviors that indicate high Learning Agility. Because behaviors are readily observable, behavioral statements can be rated by the targeted individuals and others around them. In addition, this assessment provides people with meaningful feedback. Behavioral feedback can help individuals understand the specific actions to take in developing their Learning Agility further.

During the past 10 years, thousands of employees have been assessed using the Choices™ multi-rater instrument. A summary of key research findings is highlighted in the following paragraphs.

- In the study of a sample of 217 participants from six companies (Lombardo & Eichinger, 2000), Learning Agility explained about 30% of the variance of two outcome measures—supervisor rating of performance/potential and being able to stay out of trouble.

- People with higher Learning Agility scores performed significantly better once promoted ($R^2 = .33$). Therefore, highly learning agile individuals are better able to meet the challenges of new jobs (Eichinger & Lombardo, 2004).

- In the research of a sample ($N = 107$) of law enforcement employees, Learning Agility was found to predict supervisor rating of job promotability and overall job performance over cognitive ability and personality ($\Delta R^2 = .10$ and $.06$, standardized $\beta = .32$ and $.26$, $ps < .01$; Connolly & Viswesvaran, 2002).

- Overall, Learning Agility has been found to have a normal distribution in the employee population (De Meuse, Dai, Hallenbeck, & Tang, 2008). Because companies typically administer a Learning Agility assessment to a selective group of (high potential) employees, a skewed distribution would typically be found. The distribution has a preponderance of high mean scores. When administered to a non-selective group of employees, a normal distribution of Learning Agility scores will be observed.

- In general, Learning Agility scores are unrelated to gender (De Meuse et al., 2008; Lombardo & Eichinger, 2003). However, as expected, females scored slightly higher than males on the People Agility subscale. This finding is consistent with the literature, in that females appear to be more attuned to others, learn more from others, and have more versatile interpersonal skills on average than do men. Overall, there were no statistically significant differences between males and females on *overall* Learning Agility.

- Learning Agility generally is unrelated to age (De Meuse et al., 2008). There is some evidence that younger individuals tend to score slightly higher than older ones on the Change Agility subscale (Lombardo & Eichinger, 2003). However, *overall* Learning Agility mean scores were not statistically different across age groups.

- There also is no evidence suggesting significant ethnicity-related differences on Learning Agility as assessed by the Choices™ assessment (Church, 2006; De Meuse et al., 2008).

- Data obtained from different regions of the world—North America, South America, Europe, Asia, Australia/New Zealand—reveal that the Choices™ assessment is a reliable instrument for measuring Learning Agility. Cronbach alpha reliability coefficients for the overall scale and each of the four subscales exceeded 0.85 in all five of the above global regions (De Meuse et al., 2008).

- Individuals generally lack awareness of the extent of their Learning Agility (De Meuse et al., 2008). When we placed employees into the following three groups—high potential, middle potential, and low potential— and then compared their self-ratings with others' ratings, we observed that individuals in the *low* potential group tend to *overrate* themselves. In contrast, individuals in the *high* potential group tend to *underrate* themselves. This pattern of self-other agreement is consistent with the findings on other multisource assessments (Atwater & Yammarino, 1992; Eichinger & Lombardo, 2004).

- One Fortune 500 special materials company identified approximately 100 "high potentials" through a series of talent review sessions. Subsequently, these employees were administered the Choices™ assessment. Based on the survey, nearly 70% of them were classified as "high potentials," and the remaining employees all had scores above the population mean (De Meuse et al., 2008). Thus, scores on the Choices™ assessment were highly related to an independent assessment of high potential.

- A study was conducted in seven best practice organizations in the field of talent management (Dries, Vantilborgh, & Pepermans, 2012). Learning Agility as assessed by the Choices™ assessment was found to be a better predictor of being identified as a high potential than job performance. According to the authors, high performers are three times more likely to be identified as high potentials than employees with a lower performance. However, being high in Learning Agility increases a person's likelihood of being identified as a high potential by 18 times.

- In a multiyear longitudinal study conducted in a large direct sales company operated in China, scores on the Choices™ assessment were significantly correlated with performance ratings in concurrent year ($r = .43$, $p<.01$), the first year ($r = .37$, $p<.01$), and the second year ($r = .32$, $p<.05$) after the Learning Agility assessment. In addition, Learning Agility scores predicted the number of promotions participants received over the two years ($r = .39$, $p<.01$).

THE DEVELOPMENT OF LEARNING AGILITY FOR TOMORROW'S LEADERS

Obviously, not all individuals are successful when promoted. Research consistently indicates that certain types of individuals are more likely than others to move into senior positions (Mumford, Zaccaro, Johnson, Diana, Gilbert, & Threlfall, 2000). As suggested by Charan, Drotter, and Noel (2011), the passage from lower position levels to higher levels not only requires developing new skills, it also demands that leaders break old behavioral habits and accept new values that may be contradictory with previous ones. Learning Agility appears to be a prerequisite for the successful progression up the leadership pipeline.

Given the importance of Learning Agility to leadership effectiveness, a frequently asked question is, "Can we develop a manager's Learning Agility?" And, "If yes, how do we develop a manager's Learning Agility?"

Can Learning Agility Be Developed?

Learning Agility is a relatively stable individual attribute. However, like many other individual differences such as personalities and abilities, both nature and nurture play roles in shaping where we are today. With dedication and deliberate practice, people can and do make meaningful improvements in Learning Agility. It usually starts with individuals' attitudes and values. If individuals believe that they can learn and grow, improvement is more likely to occur. But, most importantly, people can be more conscious about learning. Self-consciousness, or mindfulness, is a flexible state of mind in which we are actively engaged in the present, noticing new things, and being sensitive to context. When we are in a state of mindlessness, we behave more like pre-programmed automatons that act solely according to past behaviors. When we engage in mindful learning, we avoid forming mind-sets that unnecessarily limit us. A case articulated by McCall and Hollenbeck (2008) illustrates this point well:

> As part of a research project, one of the authors spent a year following newly promoted executives, asking two simple questions: "What did you do last week?" and "What did you learn from it?" At first, the executives had trouble remembering what they had done during all the "business" of the preceding period, much less what they might have learned. As the project went on, they began to pay more attention to what was happening, and as attention increased, became more aware of the learning that was available to them. As a result of paying attention, many of them began to try informal experiments or changed their approach just to see what would happen (p. 24).

How Does a Person Develop Learning Agility?

Individuals who are learning agile proactively seek diverse job experiences. Plus, they are more likely to learn more from those diverse experiences. But how to develop someone's Learning Agility? It is still through experience—a variety of experience.

The benefit of being specialized in a functional area is the increased level of expertise and functional and technical efficiency. However, the disadvantage associated with being specialized is the risk of becoming trapped in cognitive inflexibility. If a person spends his/her whole career in one specialized area of function, it is harder to adapt to a new specialty, new functional area, or new technology due to what Hall (1986) calls "career routine." On the other hand, diverse experience promotes flexibility and adaptability of individuals. The finding from the research is consistent. When people have a diversity of job experience, they are more learning agile (Dries, et al., 2012; Karaevli & Hall, 2006). Organizations also rate employees' promotability high when they have taken challenging job experiences. Therefore, there is a reciprocal relationship between Learning Agility and job experience. High learning agile individuals constantly look for diverse job experiences. In return, diverse job experiences reinforce ones' Learning Agility. Figure 2 depicts this reciprocal relationship. A good resource for developing Learning Agility through job experience is the book *Becoming an Agile Leader: A Guide to Learning From Your Experiences* (Orr, 2012).

Figure 2. The Reciprocal Relationship Between Learning Agility and Experience

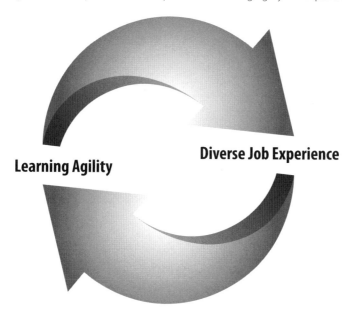

Learning Agility　　　　**Diverse Job Experience**

In addition to diverse job experiences, there are other techniques that can be used to accelerate Learning Agility development. Assessment and feedback is a development accelerator. Because Learning Agility is a multidimensional concept, not all high learning agile individuals are the same. Similarly, not all low learning agile individuals are low for the same reasons. Through assessment and feedback, a person can enhance his/her self-awareness by revealing the blind spots (areas where the person believes he/she *is more skilled* than is perceived by others) and hidden strengths (areas where the person believes he/she is *less skilled* than is perceived by others). Learning Agility is much more than just an abstract concept. It is characterized by certain behaviors and preferences. Because it's a set of behaviors, you can detect and spot these behaviors and develop these qualities by changing and learning new behaviors (Swisher, 2012). Over time, these learned behaviors can be internalized to form a sustainable personal trait—Learning Agility. Subsequent chapters in this book provide many developmental tips to help change and develop these behaviors associated with Learning Agility.

People can increase their Learning Agility through systematic and persistent efforts. Organizational leaders should recognize that employees are much more willing to challenge themselves and take risks when the company's culture fosters such a learning orientation (Senge, 1990). A learning culture encourages employees to share information, provide feedback to each other, and try innovative solutions. Consequently, organizations must establish a culture that encourages such behaviors (Ruyle, Eichinger, & De Meuse, 2009). The development of employees' Learning Agility doesn't happen coincidentally. Learning and development is less likely to occur when the organizational environment does not support it.

The development of Learning Agility also requires individuals themselves to break from habitual behavioral patterns at work. Complacency and comfortable work routines need to be avoided (Hooijberg & Quinn, 1992). Individuals must challenge and stretch themselves. New job behaviors need to be enacted. Once change is instilled as a common workplace occurrence on the job, the confidence and ability to accept new challenges increases and development occurs. Research suggests that executives learn most from hardship—job assignments at which they fail or perform poorly (Lombardo & Eichinger, 2011; McCall et al., 1988). Such incidents require individuals to be resilient, possessing the ability to manage and deal with stress effectively. If they do not, they will react by resisting, withdrawing, or burning out. Researchers of management transition and cross-cultural assignment have observed that emotional resilience is one of the critical success factors (Stahl & Caligiuri, 2005). Emotional resilience seems to be an important component of Learning Agility. For Learning Agility to develop, it seems reasonable that individuals will need to improve their emotional resilience.

CONCLUDING REMARKS

Ever since the "war for talent" was popularized by the 1997 McKinsey report, the concept of identifying and managing high potentials has become increasingly important for organizations. More than a decade later, the war for talent has still not ended. If anything, it is actually escalating! The development of the next generation of leaders can't be overstated. Perhaps we should ask what percentage of *your* senior executives are promoted internally. Pharmacy giant Medco fills nearly 80% of vice president and higher positions with internal candidates (Donlon, 2009). One of the hallmarks of 3M's culture is to view virtually every employee as a potential leader. Fully 73% of senior executives and HR leaders indicate that the urgency to develop leaders in their organizations has increased during the past three years (Donlon, 2009).

One of the tremendous advantages of using a tool like the Choices™ assessment is that it provides an independent, quantifiable assessment of an individual's potential. It provides management with an objective measure of the likelihood of success if promoted. As a *Bloomberg Businessweek* poll documented, individuals' perceptions are subject to bias. In the poll, 90% of the 2,000 executives who were asked claimed that they were in the top 10% of talent in their respective organizations (Coy, 2007). Potential needs to be determined through systematic assessment. In addition, the separate dimension scores on the Choices™ assessment enable the development of specific individual action plans to enhance the Learning Agility of an organization's workforce.

More than ever, organizations today require leaders (indeed, all employees) who are open to change, flexible, and willing to continuously learn, grow, and evolve. They need leaders who thrive on new challenges and experiences. Leaders who possess great people skills, a high tolerance for ambiguity, vision, and innovation. In short, leaders who are learning agile.

....

If you want one year of prosperity, grow grain.
If you want 10 years of prosperity, grow trees.
If you want 100 years of prosperity, grow people.

Another Chinese Proverb

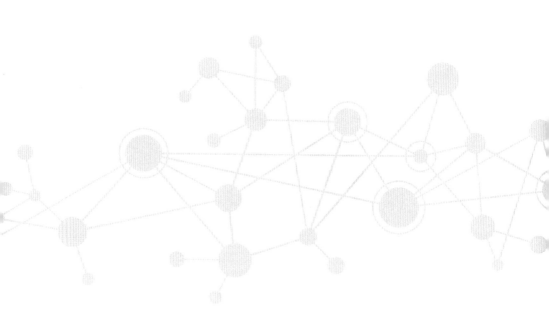

References

Arun, N., Coyle, P. T., & Hauenstein, N. (2012). Learning agility: Still searching for clarity on a confounded construct. *Industrial and Organizational Psychology, 5*(3), 290–293.

Atwater, L. E., & Yammarino, F. J. (1992). Does self-other agreement on leadership perceptions moderate the validity of leadership and performance predictions? *Personnel Psychology, 45,* 41–164.

Bennis, W. G., & Thomas, R. J. (2002). *Geeks & geezers: How era, values, and defining moments shape leaders.* Boston, MA: Harvard Business School Press.

Blanchard, K. (2007). Top challenges. *Leadership Excellence, 24*(6), 4.

Bray, D. W., Campbell, R. J., & Grant, D. L. (1974). *Formative years in business: A long-term AT&T study of managerial lives.* New York, NY: John Wiley and Sons, Inc.

Carette, B., & Anseel, F. (2012). Epistemic motivation is what gets the learner started. *Industrial and Organizational Psychology, 5*(3), 306–309.

Charan, R. (2005). Ending the CEO succession crisis. *Harvard Business Review, 83*(2), 72–81.

Charan, R., Drotter, S., & Noel, J. (2011). *The leadership pipeline: How to build the leadership powered company* (2nd ed.). San Francisco, CA: Jossey-Bass.

Church, A. H. (2006, May). *Talent management: Will the high potentials please stand up?* Symposium presented at the annual conference of the Society for Industrial and Organizational Psychology, Dallas, TX.

Connolly, J. A., & Viswesvaran, C. (2002, April). *Assessing the construct validity of a measure of learning agility.* Paper presented at the annual conference of the Society for Industrial and Organizational Psychology, Toronto, Canada.

Corporate Leadership Council. (2005). *Realizing the full potential of rising talent (Volume I): A quantitative analysis of the identification and development of high-potential employees.* Washington, DC: Corporate Executive Board.

Coy, P. (2007, August 19). Ten years from now. *Bloomberg Businessweek.* Retrieved from http://www.businessweek.com/stories/2007-08-19/ten-years-from-now-and

De Meuse, K. P., Dai, G., & Hallenbeck, G. S. (2010). Learning agility: A construct whose time has come. *Consulting Psychology Journal: Practice and Research, 62*(2), 119–130.

De Meuse, K. P., Dai, G., Hallenbeck, G., & Tang, K. (2008). *Global talent management: Using learning agility to identify high potentials around the world*. Los Angeles, CA: Korn/Ferry Institute.

De Meuse, K. P., Dai, G., Swisher, V. V., Eichinger, R. W., & Lombardo, M. M. (2012). Leadership development: Exploring, clarifying, and expanding our understanding of learning agility. *Industrial and Organizational Psychology, 5*(3), 280–286.

DeRue, D. S., Ashford, S. J., & Myers, C. G. (2012). Learning agility: In search of conceptual clarity and theoretical grounding. *Industrial and Organizational Psychology, 5*(3), 258–279.

Donlon, J. P. (2009). Best companies for leaders. *Chief Executive Magazine.* Retrieved from http://chiefexecutive.net/best-companies-for-leaders

Dries, N., Vantilborgh, T., & Pepermans, R. (2012). The role of learning agility and career variety in the identification and development of high potential employees. *Personnel Review, 41*(3), 340–358.

Dychtwald, K., Erickson, T. J., & Morison, R. (2006). *Workforce crisis: How to beat the coming shortage of skills and talent*. Boston, MA: Harvard Business School Press.

Eichinger, R. W., & Lombardo, M. M. (2004). Learning agility as a prime indicator of potential. *Human Resource Planning, 27*(4), 12–15.

Finkelstein, S. M. (2003). *Why smart executives fail: And what you can learn from their mistakes*. New York, NY: Portfolio.

Freedman, A. M. (1998). Pathways and crossroads to institutional leadership. *Consulting Psychology Journal: Practice and Research, 50*(3), 131–151.

Gehler, C. P. (2005). *Agile leaders, agile institutions: Educating adaptive and innovative leaders for today and tomorrow*. Carlisle, PA: Strategic Studies Institute, U. S. Army War College.

Goldsmith, M., & Reiter, M. (2007). *What got you here won't get you there: How successful people become even more successful*. New York, NY: Hyperion.

Hall, D. T. (1986). Dilemmas in linking succession planning to individual executive learning. *Human Resource Management, 25*(2), 235–265.

Hewitt Associates. (2005). The top companies for leaders. *Journal of the Human Resource Planning Society, 28*(3), 18–23. Retrieved from http://www.inspireimagineinnovate.com/pdf/Top_Companies_2005_Report.pdf

Hezlett, S. A., & Kuncel, N. R. (2012). Prioritizing the learning agility research agenda. *Industrial and Organizational Psychology, 5*(3), 296–301.

Hogan, R., & Kaiser, R. B. (2005). What we know about leadership. *Review of General Psychology, 9*(2), 169–180.

Hooijberg, R., & Quinn, R. E. (1992). Behavioral complexity and the development of effective managers. In R. L. Philips & J. G. Hunt (Eds.), *Strategic leadership: A multiorganizational-level perspective* (pp.161–176). New York, NY: Quorum Books.

Howard, A. (2009). *Global leader SOS: Can multinational leadership skills be developed?* Symposium presented at the annual conference of the Society for Industrial and Organizational Psychology, New Orleans, LA.

Howard, A., & Bray, D. (1988). *Managerial lives in transition: Advancing age and changing times*. New York, NY: Guilford Press.

Kaiser, R. B. (2008). *The importance, assessment, and devilment of flexible leadership*. Symposium presented at the annual conference of the Society for Industrial and Organizational Psychology, San Francisco, CA.

Kaiser, R. B., Lindberg, J. T., & Craig, S. B. (2007). Assessing the flexibility of managers: A comparison of methods. *International Journal of Selection and Assessment, 15*(1), 40–55.

Karaevli, A., & Hall, D. T. T. (2006). How career variety promotes the adaptability of managers: A theoretical model. *Journal of Vocational Behavior, 69*(3), 359–373.

Lombardo, M. M., & Eichinger, R. W. (1989). *Preventing derailment: What to do before it's too late*. Greensboro, NC: Center for Creative Leadership.

Lombardo, M. M., & Eichinger, R. W. (2000). High potentials as high learners. *Human Resource Management, 39*(4), 321–330.

Lombardo, M. M., & Eichinger, R. W. (2003). *Choices Architect® User's Manual*. Minneapolis, MN: Lominger International: A Korn/Ferry Company.

Lombardo, M. M., & Eichinger, R. W. (2011). *The leadership machine: Architecture to develop leaders for any future* (10th Anniversary ed.). Minneapolis, MN: Lominger International: A Korn/Ferry Company.

Lombardo, M. M., Ruderman, M. N., & McCauley, C. D. (1988). Explanations of success and derailment in upper-level management positions. *Journal of Business and Psychology, 2*(3), 199–216.

McCall, M. W., Jr., & Hollenbeck, G. P. (2002). *Developing global executives: The lessons of international experience*. Boston, MA: Harvard Business School Press.

McCall, M. W., Jr., & Hollenbeck, G. P. (2008). Developing the expert leader. *People & Strategy, 31*(1), 20–28.

McCall, M. W., Jr., & Lombardo, M. M. (1983). What makes a top executive? *Psychology Today, 17*(2), 26–31.

McCall, M. W., Jr., Lombardo, M. M., & Morrison, A. M. (1988). *The lessons of experience: How successful executives develop on the job.* New York, NY: Free Press.

McCauley, C. D., Ruderman, M. N., Ohlott, P. J., & Morrow, J. E. (1994). Assessing the developmental components of managerial jobs. *Journal of Applied Psychology, 79*(4), 544–560.

Morrison, A., White, R., & Van Velsor, E. (1987, rev. 1992). *Breaking the glass ceiling: Can women reach the top of America's largest corporations?* Reading, MA: Addison Wesley.

Mueller-Hanson, R. A., White, S. S., Dorsey, D. W., & Pulakos, E. D. (2005). *Training adaptable leaders: Lessons from research and practice* (Report No. 1844). Minneapolis, MN: Personnel Decisions Research Institutes.

Mumford, M. D., Zaccaro, S. J., Johnson, J. F., Diana, M., Gilbert, J. A., & Threlfall, K. V. (2000). Patterns of leader characteristics: Implications for performance and development. *Leadership Quarterly, 11*(1), 115–133.

Orr, J. E. (2012). *Becoming an agile leader: A guide to learning from your experiences.* Minneapolis, MN: Lominger International: A Korn/Ferry Company.

Pepermans, R., Vloeberghs, D., & Perkisas, B. (2003). High potential identification policies: An empirical study among Belgian companies. *Journal of Management Development, 22*(8), 660–678.

Ruyle, K. E., Eichinger, R. W., & De Meuse, K. P. (2009). *FYI™ for talent engagement: Drivers of best practice for managers and business leaders.* Minneapolis, MN: Lominger International: A Korn/Ferry Company.

Senge, P. M. (1990). *The fifth discipline: The art & practice of the learning organization.* London, England: Currency.

Slan-Jerusalim, R., & Hausdorf, P. A. (2007). Managers' justice perceptions of high potential identification practices. *Journal of Management Development, 26*(10), 933–950.

Snell, R. (1992). Experiential learning at work: Why can't it be painless? *Personnel Review, 21*(4), 12–26.

Spreitzer, G. M., McCall, M. W., Jr., & Mahoney, J. D. (1997). Early identification of international executive potential. *Journal of Applied Psychology, 82*(1), 6–29.

Stahl, G. K., & Caligiuri, P. M. (2005).The effectiveness of expatriate coping strategies: The moderating role of cultural distance, position level, and time on the international assignment. *Journal of Applied Psychology, 90*(4), 603–615.

Sternberg, R. J. (1984). *Beyond IQ: A triarchic theory of human intelligence.* New York, NY: Cambridge University Press.

Sternberg, R. J. (1997). *Successful intelligence: How practical and creative intelligence determine success in life.* New York, NY: Plume.

Sternberg, R. J., Wagner, R. K., Williams, W. W., & Horvath, J. A. (1995). Testing common sense. *American Psychologist, 50*(11), 912–927.

Swisher, V. V. (2012). *Becoming an agile leader: Know what to do…When you don't know what to do.* Minneapolis, MN: Lominger International: A Korn/Ferry Company.

Van Velsor, E., & Leslie, J. B. (1995). Why executives derail: Perspectives across time and culture. *Academy of Management Executive, 9*(4), 62–72.

Wells, S. J. (2003). Who's next? *HR Magazine, 48*(11), 44–50.

Wong, L. (2004). *Developing adaptive leaders: The crucible experience of operation Iraqi Freedom.* Carlisle, PA: Strategic Studies Institute, U. S. Army War College.

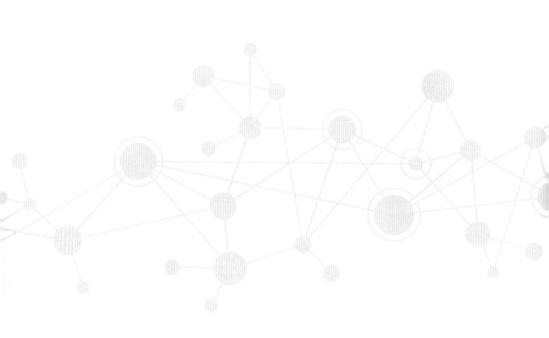

Self~Awareness

Being self-aware means knowing yourself but also understanding your impact on others and being open to making course corrections. Self-Awareness is fueled by a desire to continuously improve yourself. For individuals who are highly self-aware, investing time and energy in personal growth is a given. They are always on the lookout for new things to learn, new experiences to have, and new skills to improve. For them, even when they are presented with a challenge, a hardship, or an undesirable situation, the silver lining is finding something they can take away from that experience. Part of what helps self-aware individuals grow and change is feedback. The self-aware person views everything and everyone around them as potential sources of feedback. Not only are they able to hear critical feedback without getting defensive, they make changes based on what they heard. Feedback from others helps fuel introspection and reflection for the highly self-aware person. Playing back how an interaction unfolded and what they might have done differently is a common exercise for them. By reflecting, they are also better able to identify and articulate the thoughts and feelings behind their actions. Keeping tabs on what they're feeling and why is a critical component to maintaining their composure, even in highly stressful or emotional situations. And while self-aware individuals are clearly attuned to their strengths and weaknesses, their mistakes and shortcomings, they don't use this knowledge to beat themselves up. On the contrary, they generally stay upbeat about what's possible, even in light of challenging circumstances.

DIMENSIONS

Personal Learner

Feedback Oriented

Reflective

Emotion Management

Self-Knowledge

Personal Learner

Personal Learners view themselves as a work in progress. They are committed to the journey of self-improvement rather than a specific destination of perfection. Every experience presents them with an opportunity to learn. And when learning opportunities don't fall in their lap, they go searching for new things to learn, new skills to hone, new insights to reflect on. Along with this energetic, proactive approach to learning comes a propensity to inquire, to search for meaning and lessons: What did I do? What could I do differently? What impact did I have on people and on the situation? How might this have been seen? How might I change or adjust next time? Being a Personal Learner brings many benefits—both personally and professionally. For you personally, you have the opportunity to become a better version of yourself through constantly learning. Being an eager learner has value for you professionally as well. A demonstrated focus on continuous learning has been related to everything from sales success to level attained in organizations. Learning new skills is a prime predictor of promotion and career success.

There is nothing noble in being superior to your fellow man;
true nobility is being superior to your former self.

Lao-Tzu
Chinese philosopher (c. 6th century BCE)

SKILLED
Seeks continuous self-improvement
Motivated to add new skills to repertoire
Actively seeks new ways to grow and be challenged
Willing to weather temporary setbacks in pursuit of long-term growth

LESS SKILLED

Comfortable with current skills

Is satisfied with who they are

Doesn't put effort into growth and change

Fearful of making missteps or mistakes that accompany learning

OVERUSE OF SKILL

Focuses on self-improvement to the detriment of meeting other obligations

Susceptible to the latest self-help fad

Shows too much humility and lack of confidence regarding own strengths

Gets absorbed in learning when the situation calls for immediate action

SOME POSSIBLE CAUSES OF LOWER SKILL

Causes help explain "why" a person may have trouble in this dimension. When seeking to increase skill, it's helpful to consider how these might play out in certain situations. And remember that all of these can be addressed if you are motivated to do so.

Comfortable with what is

Doesn't take the time

Fears failure

Lacks ambition

Unwilling to admit shortcomings

Believes capability is hardwired

Low standards of excellence

Not curious

Not sure where to start

Can't handle the stress of the learning curve

DEVELOPMENTAL DIFFICULTY

When compared with other dimensions of Learning Agility, this dimension is **easier** to develop.

33

⭐ **Does It Best**

Raina Kumra[1] is in her early 30s, but her accomplished resume looks like the sum total of eight different careers. She has made a habit of growing curious about new areas, seeking out ways to build expertise, and adding new skills to her coffer. A film major, she made two documentaries and worked as a video editor. Constantly changing computer editing programs prompted her to study computer programming, which led her to interactive digital design and social media. Beyond expanding her skill base, Kumra felt compelled to explore and understand different industry sectors: she founded a non-profit, Light Up Malawi; she leads the Agency for Holistic Branding, a creative and branding firm; and she is a contractor for the U.S. government's Broadcasting Board of Governors, which oversees international media. Kumra is an intensely curious person and admits to skill hoarding. So far, her eclectic collection of skills and experiences have taken her places she never predicted.

TIPS TO INCREASE SKILL AS A PERSONAL LEARNER

Trouble prioritizing your own development?
Think first things first.

BUILD AWARENESS AND ACCEPTANCE OF YOUR DEVELOPMENT NEEDS
If you're not sure where to start, do a skills audit. First, get a good multisource assessment, a 360° questionnaire, or poll 10 people who know you well to give you detailed feedback on what you do well and not well, what they'd like to see you keep doing, start doing, and stop doing. You don't want to waste time on developing things that turn out not to be needs. Then, accept that you have a need. Don't be defensive or try to rationalize away the need. Indicate you are concerned about the need and request more detailed information so you can focus on an efficient plan for growth and development.

PICK THE RIGHT THING TO WORK ON
Identify and develop what's important. Choose wisely. Figure out what is critically important to performance in your job or success in your career. Remember that developing is about taking the long view—not just looking at fixing an immediate need, but working on what will help you in your future. This is a huge investment of your time and energy, so make sure that you're focused on something that matters to you and something that other people think is important too. Be realistic about what you can accomplish.

MAKE A PLAN AND TAKE ACTION

Create the plan. If you have accepted the need as true and you are ready to do something about it, you need three kinds of action plans. You need to know what to stop doing, start doing, and keep doing. Since you have a need in this area (you don't do this well), you need to stop some things you are doing that aren't working. In their place, you need to start doing some things you either don't like doing, haven't ever done, or don't even know about. Even if you are bad at something, there are things you do in this area that you are probably good at and should continue.

RESOURCES TO LEARN MORE

Beh, E. (2012). Powerful guidelines on effectively writing a personal development plan. *Self-Improvement Mentor*.

Gallagher, K. (2010). *Skills development for business and management students*. New York, NY: Oxford University Press.

Stuck in a rut?
Get out of your comfort zone.

GO AGAINST YOUR NATURAL GRAIN

Find an activity that goes against your natural likes and try it. For example, if you like having a detailed project plan, try working on an emerging idea for which there is no clear road map. Increase your risk tolerance. Start small so you can recover quickly. Pick a few smaller tasks or challenges and build the skill bit by bit. For example, if strategy is your development area, write a strategic plan for an initiative and show it to people to get feedback, then write a second draft. Devise a strategy for turning one of your hobbies (i.e., photography) into a business.

STRETCH YOURSELF

Try some stretching tasks, but start small. Seventy percent of skills development happens on the job. As you talk with others while building this skill, get them to brainstorm tasks and activities you can try. Write down five tasks you will commit to doing, tasks like initiate three conversations, make peace with someone you've had problems with, write a business plan for your unit, negotiate a purchase, make a speech, find something to fix. You can try tasks off the job as well: teach someone to read, be a volunteer, join a study group, take up a new hobby—whatever will help you practice your need in a fairly low-risk way. After each task, write down the positive and negative aspects of your performance and note things you will try to do better or differently next time.

 Be careful to take on the right amount of challenge. Go for an assignment that is difficult but within reach for you. Stretching yourself too far can set you up for disappointment and make you more hesitant to take on a challenge next time.

TEST YOURSELF OUT

Work to gain knowledge and experience in areas which are new and untested for you. Until you are exposed to certain experiences and situations which require a particular skill, your skill level and potential ability in that skill remain a mystery. Keep in mind, since you have never used the skill before, the most likely outcome is that you will be somewhere between low and average. Gradually increase the stakes to continually develop the skill. Don't get discouraged if it takes awhile or feels frustrating—this is what it's like to be a beginner. Be realistic in your expectations. And continue to seek both challenge and support as you try out untested areas.

RESOURCES TO LEARN MORE

Kopp, W. (2011, January 20). Advice for social entrepreneurs [Video file]. Stanford Technology Ventures Program.

Kouzes, J. M., & Posner, B. Z. (1999). *The leadership challenge planner: An action guide to achieving your personal best.* San Francisco, CA: Jossey-Bass/Pfeiffer Publishers.

Ready to broaden your horizon?
Let go and open up to new possibilities.

EXPERIMENT AND MAKE MISTAKES

You can speed up the learning process by being willing to experiment and make mistakes. Do quick experiments and trials and learn from the results. Don't expect to get it right the first time. This leads to safe and stale solutions. Many studies show that the second or third try is when we really understand the underlying dynamics of problems. To increase learning, shorten your act and get feedback loops—aiming to make them as immediate as possible. The more frequent the cycles, the more opportunities to learn; if we do something in each of three days instead of one thing every three days, we triple our learning opportunities and increase our chances of finding the right answer. Be more willing to experiment. View mistakes as part of the learning process.

LEARN FROM OTHERS

Seek out role models. Access great minds like John Stuart Mill on problem solving, or read a biography about U.S. presidents Lyndon Johnson or Ronald Reagan to learn about persuasion. Find three people who are excellent at something you want to develop in. Observe them, interview them, and see what they do that you do not. Ask them to think through an issue with you, what questions they would ask, and what they think good sources of knowledge are.

EMBRACE THE LEARNING CURVE

Keep a philosophical attitude about your learning experience. Notice how you're feeling. Are you frustrated? Do you want to quit? Acknowledge that this is just a normal stage within the learning curve. It's easy to have an eager, positive attitude at the beginning of learning something new; the challenge is sticking with it when, in reality, it's harder than you expected. Push through the discouragement and things will get better with more practice and experience. Consider keeping a learning journal. Reflecting on past learning experiences can help you keep your current growing pains in perspective.

RESOURCES TO LEARN MORE

Buxton, B. (2011). Always be a beginner. Business Innovation Factory.

Grant-Halvorson, H. (2011, February 1). Why letting yourself make mistakes means making fewer of them. *Psychology Today*.

ASSIGNMENTS TO PRACTICE SKILL

Take on an assignment so complex that it makes your head spin. This might mean increased responsibility, competing priorities, or working outside your area of expertise. Once you become aware of your personal limits, you can find ways to improve and get beyond them.

Learn something new. Shadow an expert, go back to school, build a new skill. By formally studying something new and taking time to reflect, you are more aware of what you know and what you don't know.

Manage a group or a team of people who are towering experts in something you are not. Focus on what you can learn from other people.

TAKE TIME TO REFLECT...
Here are some questions to reflect on as you focus on being a Personal Learner. Think about how you might answer these today and how, through using the tips in this chapter, you might achieve a better result in the future.

When have you been close to a goal, only to give up because you had not yet reached it? What would it have taken for you to put forth the extra effort at the time? How might your life be different today? What did you learn from this experience?

What is one thing you would like to start improving today?
What actions will you take? What will you commit to doing differently or more/less of beginning today to sustain the improvement?

In what ways have you limited your personal development?
Where would you benefit from expanding or improving your skills?
What will you commit to do in order to move toward this?

How noble and good everyone could be if, every evening
before falling asleep, they were to recall to their minds the events
of the whole day and consider exactly what has been good and bad.
Then without realizing it, you try to improve yourself
at the start of each new day.

Anne Frank
German author and Holocaust victim

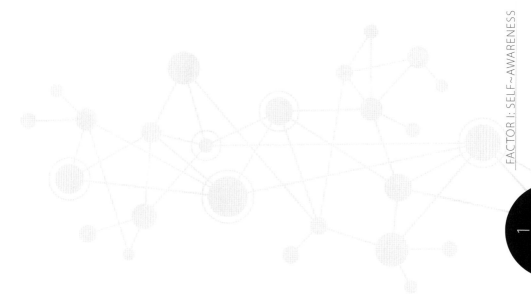

Feedback
Oriented

2

Feedback does not have to occur in a formal, sit-down conversation that starts with the phrase, "I have some feedback for you…" We encounter feedback every day, all day long—a glance in the mirror getting ready for work, an impatient response from a child or spouse, a business proposal denied approval, a thank you note from a colleague. When you are Feedback Oriented, you are an astute observer of this type of indirect feedback. You actively seek out direct feedback—both positive and constructive, and you learn from it. You know how valuable it is to get an honest read on how you are doing, what's working, and what you need to adjust. As a Feedback Oriented person, you cultivate honest relationships with others who are more than willing to share their feedback in part because it is thoughtfully considered rather than dismissed. So what makes Feedback Oriented people so good at responding to critical feedback without getting defensive? Typically, you view feedback as an opportunity for refinement, self-betterment, and becoming more effective with others. With this mind-set, and an ability to keep feedback in perspective, it becomes possible to take a more relaxed, honest look at yourself from other people's perspectives. The threats are removed but the benefits remain.

Why is it so hard to lead yourself? The answer, in my experience, lies in the differences between your idealized self—how you see yourself and how you want to be seen—and your real self. The key to growing as a leader is to narrow that gap by developing a deep self-awareness that comes from straight feedback and honest exploration of yourself, followed by a concerted effort to make changes.

Bill George
American Harvard Business School professor, former CEO of Medtronic, and author of *True North*

SKILLED
Seeks feedback and acts on it
Comfortable with personal change
Views criticism as helpful
Uses many sources for feedback
Puts feedback into perspective
Probes feedback for more understanding

LESS SKILLED
Closed, low interest in feedback or change

Doesn't voluntarily take in feedback

Denies or minimizes mistakes and shortcomings

Is seen as self-important or aloof

Takes feedback too personally

Makes excuses and blames others

OVERUSE OF SKILL
Won't take action before consulting with others

Overcorrects or overcompensates to the point of losing what makes him/her unique

Focuses too much on pleasing people

Fixates on constructive feedback or criticism

Comes across as insecure or too needy for feedback

SOME POSSIBLE CAUSES OF LOWER SKILL
Causes help explain "why" a person may have trouble in this dimension. When seeking to increase skill, it's helpful to consider how these might play out in certain situations. And remember that all of these can be addressed if you are motivated to do so.

Avoids conflict

Takes a victim point of view

Doesn't see any need for improvement

Defensive

Doesn't listen

Doesn't trust others

Hard to approach

Sees feedback as judgmental

Rigid or inflexible

Scared of what he/she may hear

Not goal oriented

DEVELOPMENTAL DIFFICULTY
When compared with other dimensions of Learning Agility, this dimension is **_easier_** to develop.

41

⭐ **Does It Best**

Early on in her writing career, Maya Angelou joined the Harlem Writers Guild. But she nearly quit after her first reading. She read her play *One Life. One Love.* She recalls, "Even as I read, I knew the drama was bad, but maybe someone would have lied a little." The feedback was harsh. Other members were accustomed to the exchange of blunt, constructive feedback. Angelou was not. At first, she could not move from her seat. By the end of the evening, Angelou recovered and resolved to read the group a new short story in two months' time.[2] Seeking out and responding to feedback had a guiding effect for Angelou. When a vocal instructor criticized her singing technique, she hired him as her coach. When parenting dilemmas arose, her close male friends would give her blunt feedback about how to raise her son. The feedback Angelou welcomed not only honed her abilities, it shaped who she is today.

TIPS TO INCREASE SKILL IN FEEDBACK ORIENTED

Not getting any feedback?
Ask for some.

CHECK IN WITH THOSE AROUND YOU

People are almost as reluctant to give feedback as they are to receive it. One way to get some informal feedback is to state what you already think about your behavior and see if your hunch checks out with those around you. "I think I rushed the concluding remarks a bit, did it seem that way to you?" Or, "I'm afraid I may have alienated some folks, what do you think?" This informal, open-ended check-in can be just the invitation your colleagues, boss, or direct reports need to muster the courage to give you their point of view.

ASK FOR MORE SPECIFICS

If you need clarity on some feedback that you've received, ask for more specifics. It's important to do this in a non-threatening, non-defensive way, otherwise people will just clam up or retract the original feedback. Tell them that you are interested in understanding more deeply because you really want to figure out what needs to change. Ask them what they would like to see you keep doing, start doing, stop doing, or do differently. If you know the people well, you can try face-to-face feedback, although you should know that this is usually blander and more positive than written feedback. If you do this, select specific areas and state what you think the issue or need for improvement is. Don't ask general questions. Get them to respond to the specific areas you want to explore.

PARTICIPATE IN A FORMAL 360° MULTI-RATER ASSESSMENT

People who don't know their strengths and weaknesses tend to overestimate themselves. This is a consistent finding in the research literature and has been related to both poor performance and being terminated. 360° feedback, where you compare your responses on a set of behaviors to those of boss, peers, direct reports (if any), and sometimes customers, is a more formal way to get honest feedback. The feedback is compiled and shared in a way that maintains anonymity (aside from the boss), which helps feedback providers be candid. And it helps you to begin to understand others' perceptions of your skills.

RESOURCES TO LEARN MORE

Bell, M. (2012). Why you need to ask for feedback from others. *Business Know-How*.

Donnelly, T. (2010, August 10). How to get feedback from employees. *Inc.com*

Not sure how to receive feedback?
View feedback as a gift.

SHOW YOUR OPENNESS TO FEEDBACK

It takes courage to give feedback. Be respectful of the person providing the feedback, acknowledge the feedback, and thank them for it. Any signal that you are closed to feedback—checking your watch, pursing your lips, looking distracted or too busy—will shut down this and future conversations. And, regardless of the feedback, accept it. Don't say it's inaccurate or a one-time failing; don't argue or qualify. Just take it in. Use mental rehearsal to get ready for what may happen. If you comment at all, give examples of the behavior being described to validate what they are saying. An open response encourages more feedback over time.

GET FOCUSED, NOT DEFENSIVE

When you receive formal feedback, focus on the highest and lowest ratings from each group. Don't spend time worrying about whether your scores are high or low compared to other people. For development, you should focus on relative scores. What are your highest and lowest ratings? Also, don't try to figure out who said what so that you can explain away the feedback. Take the energy you would spend defending and put it toward understanding and figuring out ways to continuously improve.

REFLECT ON ROOT CAUSES

Thinking about the root of the issue can be helpful in determining an action plan. Ask why: Why am I seen this way? How did my strengths get to be so? Are my weaknesses things I avoid, things I am simply not skilled at, things I dislike or things I've never done? What experiences shaped my pattern? Do I have strengths that are related to my weaknesses, such as the smart person who makes others feel less so? Use this analysis to determine what is relatively easier and tougher for you to do and why that's the case.

 Be careful not to dwell too long on why you got certain feedback or how people perceive you. If you are too hard on yourself every time you get some feedback, you will be less likely to view it as a way to continuously improve. You might start dreading it. Others will pick up on your apprehension and cut back on their efforts to provide feedback.

RESOURCES TO LEARN MORE

Heathfield, S. M. (2012). Receive feedback with grace and dignity. *About.com*

Lore, M. J. (2010). *Managing thought: Think differently. Think powerfully. Achieve new levels of success.* New York, NY: McGraw-Hill.

Not sure how to respond to feedback?
Commit to doing something with it.

CHANGE PEOPLE'S PERCEPTIONS

Feedback is subjective but it is also valid. Even if you disagree with someone's perception, you still need to address their feedback. Show your true intent through action. If people, especially those above you, continue to have misperceptions about you, your career will be damaged. You need to construct a plan to change their perception by deeds, not words. Plan how you will act in critical situations, and expect it to take quite a while for people to see you differently. It may take eight times before people reconsider their view of you.

DISCLOSE MORE

Some people think expressing doubt shows weakness. If you deny, minimize, or excuse away shortcomings, take a chance and admit that you're imperfect like everyone else. Research shows that people's perception of you improves when you simply disclose you have skill gaps and are looking to improve. Let your inside thoughts out in the open more often. Sprinkle normal work conversation with doubts, what you're thinking about, and what's getting in the way. Since you probably don't know how to do this, select three people who are good at admitting mistakes and shortcomings and observe how they do it. Not only does this humanize you, people will perceive you as someone who is willing to accept feedback.

OWN YOUR MISTAKES

Take responsibility for your mistakes. Admit mistakes matter-of-factly, inform everyone potentially affected, learn from it so the mistake isn't repeated, then move on. Take the opportunity to laugh at yourself a little bit. A little self-deprecation works wonders. Dwelling on the past is useless. Build up your heat shield. Successful people make lots of mistakes. Being right much more than two-thirds of the time is impossible if you're doing anything new. Don't let the possibility of being wrong keep you from standing up and trying. Mistakes are a rich source of feedback and present great—if sometimes painful—learning opportunities.

RESOURCES TO LEARN MORE

George, B. (2007). *True north: Discover your authentic leadership.* San Francisco, CA: Jossey-Bass.

Houlihan, M. (2012, September 21). Oops, my bad! 5 Ways your business can improve by admitting to mistakes. *Entrepreneur.*

ASSIGNMENTS TO PRACTICE SKILL

Work outside of your home country and culture. Whether you relocate, manage a global team, or interview customers from different regions, use the opportunity to build awareness of how you can be more effective in varied contexts.

Become a student. Build new skills and expertise. No matter how accomplished you are in certain areas, it can be advantageous to remember what it's like to be a beginner. Notice the feedback you get along the way as you move through the learning curve.

Attend a leadership development course or workshop that includes 360° and/or live feedback. Take time to reflect on the feedback. Notice your first reaction and how you process both positive and constructive feedback.

TAKE TIME TO REFLECT...

Here are some questions to reflect on as you focus on being Feedback Oriented. Think about how you might answer these today and how, through using the tips in this chapter, you might achieve a better result in the future.

How well do you really know how others perceive you? How do you gather and assess information related to how others see you? What steps can you take to build ways of seeking feedback into your daily routine?

When have you focused energy on criticism to the exclusion of praise?
Or when have you ignored all the positive feedback because of one negative statement?
How can you focus constructive criticism from the perception of growing and developing?
How will you balance listening to areas for improvement with your known strengths?

Where do you tend to go for guidance and feedback? Where is their perspective strong? Where might you be missing important viewpoints? How can you expand your network to get a broader perspective? Who will you begin to include?

....

Most enjoyable activities are not natural;
they demand an effort that initially one is reluctant to make.
But once the interaction starts to provide feedback to the person's
skills, it usually begins to be intrinsically rewarding.

Mihaly Csikszentmihalyi
Hungarian professor of psychology, leading expert in positive psychology, and author of *Flow*

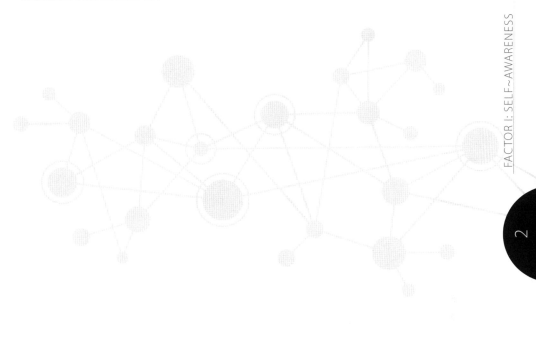

Reflective

Being Reflective is at the heart of being a learner. No matter what you call it—mindfulness, being present, living consciously, purposefulness—cultivating a Reflective mind-set requires the time, the space, and the desire to sit with and examine your thoughts, feelings, and actions. It is through reflection that you make sense of your experiences, take lessons from those experiences, and make adjustments for the future. You might begin to reflect by looking back at a situation and asking yourself, "What impact did I have? What could I have done differently?" But reflection doesn't only take place after the fact. You can be Reflective in the midst of an interaction while the situation is still unfolding. Notice how an increase in observing and reflecting often slows things down and leads to breakthroughs.

I think before I act—and then think again. I am not entirely a coward, but I do not lose myself in action as you do.

John Christopher
Pseudonym for Christopher Samuel Youd, British science fiction author

SKILLED
Learns from mistakes
Takes time and makes space for introspection
Is able to explain rationale behind actions and decisions
Contemplates what he/she could have done differently
Reflects back on his/her impact on others and situations
Knows what causes his/her feelings and moods

3

LESS SKILLED
Acts impulsively

Struggles to articulate the *why* behind decisions, feelings, or actions

Doesn't look back

Rationalizes past mistakes

OVERUSE OF SKILL
Gets stuck in the past

Is overly self-critical

Is overly self-conscious of thoughts and feelings

Self-checks so much that things don't get done

Favors thinking over action

SOME POSSIBLE CAUSES OF LOWER SKILL
Causes help explain "why" a person may have trouble in this dimension. When seeking to increase skill, it's helpful to consider how these might play out in certain situations. And remember that all of these can be addressed if you are motivated to do so.

Rushed

Distracted

Defensive

Needs to be right

Arrogant

Too much success

In denial

Avoids accountability

DEVELOPMENTAL DIFFICULTY
When compared with other dimensions of Learning Agility, this dimension is **easier** to develop.

Did You Know?

Being more reflective makes you more effective. Recent research by the Center for Creative Leadership (CCL) in partnership with Teachers College of Columbia University shows that leaders who are rated low on reflectiveness are considered to be less effective by their peers and direct reports. And, while reflection is not in and of itself a difficult thing to do, a recent poll conducted by CCL shows that 24% of respondents think that being reflective is one of the most challenging things to do on the job.[3]

TIPS TO INCREASE SKILL IN BEING REFLECTIVE

Too busy to clear your mind?
Take a time out.

TAKE A BREAK
Find something non-verbal to do. The left side of your brain may get more of a workout during the work day. Don't forget to feed the non-verbal side. If you're busy solving problems and don't think you have time to take a break, consider this: research shows that breakthroughs happen when we are not focused directly on solving the problem. Sleeping, swimming, yoga, walking, or doing something creative can all provide the space for our brain to work things out on its own.

FIND SOME PEACE
Maybe you have a favorite park or path. Maybe there is a particular landmark or lookout that helps you feel grounded. Find a place that puts you in a reflective frame of mind. Take a drive. Hop on your bike. Find a retreat center. Walk a labyrinth. Let your mind unwind. Reflecting can renew your energy and prepare you for whatever is next. Put on your favorite music. Find artists that use poetry, imagery, and stories in a way that speaks to you. If you haven't listened to any new artists lately, create a new station for yourself using one of the many online music libraries. Experiment with listening to music at work. Does the classical or jazz station inspire some new thinking on a project you've been working on?

MANAGE STRESS
When you're under pressure or stress, it's harder to step away from what's comfortable. In stress mode, we go to habits more readily, which stops us from taking new actions. Why? For us to be able to integrate new information properly, things have to be relatively quiet in the brain. In the research on executive derailment, making decisions under intense pressure often led

the executives to preemptively land (incorrectly) on a favorite past solution. Find ways to manage your stress levels. Give your mind clear and repetitious breakpoints—for instance, between work and non-work stressors. Signal work is over by playing music in your car, immediately play with your kids, go for a walk, swim for 20 minutes. At work, worry about work things, not life things. When you hit the driveway, worry about life things and leave work things at the office.

RESOURCES TO LEARN MORE

Stamos-Kovacs, J. (2012). Blissing out: 10 Relaxation techniques to reduce stress on-the-spot. *WebMD.*

Yager, J. (2012). *Work less, do more: The 14-day productivity makeover* (2nd ed.). Stamford, CT: Hannacroix Creek Books, Inc.

Struggling with how to reflect?
Find and use reflection tools.

CONDUCT YOUR OWN AFTER ACTION REVIEWS

Companies often conduct formal after action reviews after a project. There's no reason you can't use the same method after people interactions, decisions made, wins, losses, and so on. Have a set of questions that you reflect on: What happened? Why did it happen? What worked? Didn't work? What could I do differently next time? After you've done enough of these, you're likely to surface insights—common themes across several situations. These insights can then become lessons, principles, rules of thumb that you can use going forward.

KEEP A JOURNAL

Maybe you've tried this before. Many of us have a number of half-used notebooks where we started journals with good intentions but never followed through. Try something different this time. There are many options available these days. Maybe you can keep it with your calendar or maybe you'd rather keep a tiny notebook handy in your front pocket to capture epiphanies before they slip away. You could also use the notes app on your mobile device or an online journal.

FIND A THOUGHT-PROVOKING BOOK

There are many books out there with daily installments of thought-provoking stories, insights, or meditations. Find one that appeals to you and keep it on your nightstand or next to your favorite chair. Flag the pages that are meaningful for you and come back to them periodically. See how your thinking evolves as you take more time to ponder a given topic.

RESOURCES TO LEARN MORE

Goodreads. (2012). Popular thought provoking books. *Goodreads.com*

McFarlane, E., & Saywell, J. (1995). *If... (Questions for the game of life)* (Vol. 1). New York, NY: Villard Books.

Concerned you won't make the time?
Rely on people and plans that encourage reflection.

PUT TIME ON YOUR CALENDAR

Make reflection accessible and habitual. Once you find the practices and prompts that help you reflect, keep them close by. Keep your journal in your commuter bag. Leave the daily meditations book with thought-provoking quotes on your nightstand. Add reflection reminders to your repeating tasks. Carve out space in your home and carve out space on your calendar. Then protect it. And, remember, to form a new habit, you need to repeat it at least eight times before it sticks.

FIND A THOUGHT PARTNER WHO HELPS YOU REFLECT

This could be a colleague, a boss, a spouse, a personal coach, a long-distance friend, or even your monthly book club. Notice the people in your life who ask you good questions that make you stop and think. Then seek those people out. Ask them to have lunch, give them a call, offer your own thought-provoking questions in return. These naturally forming coaching relationships can provide support and direction for both personal and career matters.

 Reflecting on your own or with others has its benefits. But when taking time to process things is outweighing the time you spend taking action and making progress, it's time to rebalance.

INTEGRATE REFLECTION INTO YOUR LIFE

Reflection doesn't have to be a big agenda item. Keep it simple and make it part of your daily life. Do you have a favorite bookstore? Show up on the night they have an author reading. Do you spend a little time each day surfing the Internet? Look up an artist or poet who inspires you and watch an online video clip of a poem, song, or reading. Trying to plan a night out with friends? Suggest a play at a local theater, a concert, or an independent film. Pepper your life with things that make you think. Reflection will become second nature.

RESOURCES TO LEARN MORE

Addison, M., & Pavelich, K. (2012, March 20). Embracing our perfect imperfect selves [Video file]. TEDxThunderBay.

Paul, R., & Elder, L. (2001). *Critical thinking in everyday life: 9 Strategies.* The Foundation for Critical Thinking.

3

ASSIGNMENTS TO PRACTICE SKILL

Manage a team for the first time, or manage a difficult or disengaged team. Use the opportunity to reflect on your own and with others about the team dynamics and the effectiveness of your leadership of the team.

Take on a task or assignment that is brand new for you. Remind yourself of what it feels like to be a beginner. Reflect on and notice what you are experiencing as you go through each stage of the learning curve.

Work outside of your home country or culture. Reflect on your own cultural biases and perceptions and how you are making adjustments that are appropriate in this unfamiliar context.

TAKE TIME TO REFLECT...

Here are some questions to reflect on as you focus on being Reflective. Think about how you might answer these today and how, through using the tips in this chapter, you might achieve a better result in the future.

As you reflect back on your career, what experiences were most meaningful? What stands out the most? What did you learn about yourself from these experiences? What do you do differently today?

When was the last time something made you pause and reflect? How can you become more mindful about what you are reading or doing? What prevents you from pausing and reflecting about what you do, read, or observe? What will you commit to do differently?

As much as we get to know and learn about ourselves, there is much that remains unknown. What patterns of thought or behavior seem to appear without explanation? When do you find yourself asking, "Why do I keep doing this?" Where might you benefit from further exploration and reflection?

....

Life can only be understood backwards; but it must be lived forwards.

Søren Kierkegaard
Danish philosopher, theologian, poet, social critic, and religious author

Emotion
Management

Emotions are electricity and chemistry. They are designed to help you cope with emergencies and threats. They trigger predictable body changes. Emotions are designed to help us with the so-called fight or flight response—to either fight or flee from that saber-toothed tiger that could be lurking behind the next tree. Emotions temporarily make the body faster and stronger—but at a price. An emotional response decreases resources for the stomach (that's why we get upset stomachs under stress) and the thinking brain (that's why we say and do dumb things under stress). Even though we might be able to lift a heavy object off a trapped person, we can't think of the right thing to say in a tense meeting. And once the emotional response is triggered, it has to run its course. It takes 45–60 seconds to subside in most people. That's why your grandmother told you to count to 10. Trouble is, in today's modern world, the saber-toothed tiger is still a danger, but now it's in your head. Now, mere thoughts often trigger an emotional response. Events which are certainly not physically threatening, like being criticized, can set it off. Even worse, today people have added a third "f" to the fight or flight response—freeze. Emotions can shut you down and leave you speechless, neither choosing to fight (argue, respond) nor flee (calmly shut down the transaction and exit). And when you're in those emotion-ruled modes, one mode you definitely won't be in is learning mode. By understanding and managing emotional reactions, you'll learn to be cool under pressure and be able to keep your thinking brain online.

Always behave like a duck—keep calm and unruffled on the surface, but paddle like the devil underneath.

Jacob M. Braude
Author of *Braude's Treasury of Wit and Humor for All Occasions*

4

SKILLED

Stays composed under pressure and stress

Keeps frustration, anxiety, and anger in check when interacting with others

Maintains a positive, proactive attitude, despite troubling circumstances or obstacles

Is a calming presence

Weighs emotions when making decisions

Pauses before reacting

Is aware of his/her emotional triggers

LESS SKILLED

Is easily swayed by his/her emotions

Tends to escalate emotionally tense situations

Gets easily overwhelmed and stressed under pressure

Is seen as unpredictable, cynical, or moody

OVERUSE OF SKILL

Shows little emotion; overly stoic

Fails to show emotion in appropriate circumstances

Buries emotions deep inside

Has a hard time empathizing with others' feelings

SOME POSSIBLE CAUSES OF LOWER SKILL

Causes help explain "why" a person may have trouble in this dimension. When seeking to increase skill, it's helpful to consider how these might play out in certain situations. And remember that all of these can be addressed if you are motivated to do so.

Defensive

Easily overwhelmed; very emotional

Lacks self-confidence

Perfectionist

Sensitive

Too much going on

Very control oriented

Weak impulse control

DEVELOPMENTAL DIFFICULTY

When compared with other dimensions of Learning Agility, this dimension is **harder** to develop.

🔍 Did You Know?

Leadership skills that involve emotions are some of the toughest areas to improve upon. This is because emotions come from our brain's limbic system. The limbic system has been designed over thousands of years to help humans respond to threats and stay safe. Once your limbic system senses a threat, you have a few options. You can express the emotion, which may not always be appropriate or well-received. You can suppress the emotion, which may turn the stress inward and show up on your health charts later. Or you can take some conscious control of the situation by noticing what you're feeling, calling it out, exploring why, and reframing your reaction. This third option helps the more highly evolved part of your brain, the prefrontal cortex, wield more influence on your reactions and decisions.

TIPS TO INCREASE SKILL IN EMOTION MANAGEMENT

Agitated on a regular basis?
Control yourself.

WATCH FOR YOUR TRIGGER POINTS/BUTTONS

Write down the last five times you lost your composure. Most people who have composure problems have three to five repeating triggers. Criticism. Loss of control. A certain kind of person. An enemy. Being surprised. Spouse. Children. Money. Authority. Try to group 90% of the events into three to five categories. Once you have the groupings, ask yourself why these are a problem. Is it ego? Losing face? Being caught short? Being found out? Causing you more work? In each grouping, what would be a more mature response? Mentally and physically rehearse a better response. Try to decrease by 10% a month the number of times you lose your composure.

CONTROL YOUR IMPULSES

People say and do inappropriate things when they lose their composure. The problem is that they say or do the first thing that occurs to them. Research shows that, generally, somewhere between the second and third thing you think of to say or do is the best option. Practice holding back your first response long enough to think of a second. When you can do that, wait long enough to think of a third before you choose. By that time, 50% of your composure problems should go away.

It's one thing to be in control of your reaction, it's another to miss an opportunity to let people know how you feel. Not showing your emotion can sometimes be perceived as stoic, cold, or even passive. Let it out (appropriately) when it can help move a situation or interaction in the right direction.

PAUSE

Our thinking and judgment are not at their best during the emotional response. Create and practice delaying tactics. Jot down a note in the margin. Go get a cup of coffee. Ask a question and listen. Go up to the flip chart and write something. Take notes. See yourself in a setting you find calming. Excuse yourself to go to the bathroom. You need about a minute to regain your composure after the emotional response is triggered. Don't do or say anything until the minute has passed.

RESOURCES TO LEARN MORE

Bregman, P. (2010, June 10). The no-drama rule of management. *Harvard Business Review.*

Graham, C. (2010, April 2). Be well at work, learn to pause . . . erase that blur! *Corporate Wellness Magazine.*

4

Making assumptions and adding meaning?
Stay objective.

DON'T TAKE THINGS PERSONALLY

Do you feel a need to punish the people and groups that set you off? Do you become hostile, angry, sarcastic, or vengeful? While all that may be temporarily satisfying to you, they will all backfire and you will lose in the long-term. A number of alternative approaches are more productive. When someone attacks you, rephrase it as an attack on a problem. Reverse the argument—ask what they would do if they were in your shoes. When the other side takes a rigid position, don't reject it. Ask why—what are the principles behind the offer, how do we know it's fair, what's the theory of the case. Play out what would happen if their position was accepted. Let the other side vent frustration, blow off steam, but don't react.

KEEP PERSPECTIVE

When you do reply to an attack, keep it to the facts and the impact on you. It's fine for you to draw conclusions about the impact on yourself ("I felt blindsided"). It's not fine for you to tell others their motives ("You blindsided me" means you did it, probably meant to, and I know the meaning of your behavior). So state the meaning for yourself; ask others what their actions meant. By stating how you feel and what you need, you help the other person avoid getting defensive. This is a much more efficient strategy for being heard and solving the problem, which was your goal in the first place.

DON'T JUMP TO CONCLUSIONS

Take quick action? Don't like ambiguity and uncertainty and act to wipe it out? Solutions first, understanding second? Take the time to really define the problem. Let people finish. Try not to interrupt. Don't finish others' sentences.

4

Ask clarifying questions. Restate the problem in your own words to everyone's satisfaction. Ask them what they think. Throw out trial solutions for debate. Then decide.

RESOURCES TO LEARN MORE

Cain, M. (2011, October 13). Don't take this personally, but you take things too personally. *Forbes.*

Muzio, E. (2011, January 26). The ladder of inference creates bad judgment [Video file].

Easily triggered?
Release some of the pressure.

GET MOVING

Find a release for your pent-up emotions. Get a physical hobby. Start an exercise routine. Jog. Walk. Chop wood. Sometimes people who have flare tempers hold it in too much, the pressure builds, and the teakettle blows. The body stores energy. It has to go somewhere. Work on releasing your work frustration off-work.

MONITOR YOUR PRESSURE GAUGE

Maybe your fuse is too long. You may wait and wait, let the pressure build, keep your concerns to yourself, then explode as a pressure release. Write down what you're concerned about, then talk about the issues with confidantes and coworkers before you blow up. If the pressure interferes with your thought processes at work (you're supposed to be listening but you're fretting instead), pick a time to worry. Say to yourself, "I'll write this down, then think about it on the way home. "Train yourself to stay in the present.

FIND THE FUN IN IT

Find the fun in everyday events and stressful situations. Don't take situations or yourself too seriously. Rather than reverting to impatience or annoyance, see if you can find some humor in it first. Laugh a little. Think about the masters of comedy—they take everyday observations and find something humorous in them. It's a matter of tuning in to and using what is around you to lighten the mood.

RESOURCES TO LEARN MORE

Goodman, J. (1995). *Laffirmations: 1001 Ways to add humor to your life and work.* Deerfield Beach, FL: Health Communications, Inc.

Mayo Clinic Staff. (2012, July 21). Exercise and stress: Get moving to manage stress. Mayo Clinic.

ASSIGNMENTS TO PRACTICE SKILL

Manage a group through a significant business crisis. Practice being a calming presence for others.

Handle a tough negotiation with an internal or external client or customer. No matter how much pressure you feel, maintaining your poker face can help you reach a good result.

Manage a dissatisfied internal or external customer; troubleshoot a performance or quality problem with a product or service. The tension may escalate, which will test your ability to keep your frustration in check.

TAKE TIME TO REFLECT...

Here are some questions to reflect on as you focus on Emotion Management. Think about how you might answer these today and how, through using the tips in this chapter, you might achieve a better result in the future.

In what situations do you find yourself the most frustrated at work? What contributes to the frustration? How do you typically respond? How effective are the typical outcomes? What would you like to do differently in these situations in the future?

Where have your feelings or emotions gotten in the way of your better judgment? How have feelings impaired your ability to evaluate facts in the past? What can you do to ensure you base your decisions more on intellect than emotion?

Think about a recent time when you received criticism or had your feelings hurt. What was your role in the situation? How did your perceptions of the event affect how you felt? How might your interpretation of the information have changed the way you felt about it?

A lady must retain always her composure.
Even in a rainstorm, she must appear joyous and dry.
When she loses her composure, then the respect of her peers and
her staff will follow in short order.

Anna Godbersen
American writer and author of young adult fiction

5

Self-Knowledge

People who don't know their strengths and weaknesses tend to overestimate themselves, a consistent finding in the research literature that has been related to both poor performance and being terminated. On the other hand, knowing yourself helps you use your strengths better, compensate for what you're not good at, develop where you can, and substitute skills for areas where you are unskilled. Most of us need a coach or a colleague to help us think things through, to become aware of our helpful and not-so-helpful behaviors, accept our strengths and weaknesses, and recognize the impact we have on others. As a self-aware individual, you often fulfill the coaching role for yourself. You take a proactive approach to self-insight. Being high in Self-Knowledge means that you are also very open with others about your weaknesses, shortcomings, and mistakes. You are realistic about your strengths and your development needs. And you know how your approach, style, and skill set affects other people around you. Because you are straight with yourself and straightforward with others, you tend to be regarded as a transparent, grounded, and authentic leader—qualities that typically engender other people's trust.

A moment's insight is sometimes worth a life's experience.

Oliver Wendell Holmes
American Associate Justice of the Supreme Court of the United States

SKILLED

Knows own strengths and weaknesses

Admits to mistakes and shortcomings

Is not surprised by negative or constructive feedback

Admits when he/she doesn't know

Enjoys experiences that lead to deeper self-insight

LESS SKILLED

Has unrealistic expectations for himself/herself

Doesn't acknowledge his/her limits

Is out of touch with how he/she is perceived by others

Tends to overestimate or underestimate his/her performance and contribution

OVERUSE OF SKILL

Is too open about shortcomings

Is too focused on gaining self-insight

Is too self-critical

Is overly self-conscious about his/her impact on others

SOME POSSIBLE CAUSES OF LOWER SKILL

Causes help explain "why" a person may have trouble in this dimension. When seeking to increase skill, it's helpful to consider how these might play out in certain situations. And remember that all of these can be addressed if you are motivated to do so.

Blames others for own faults

Defensive

Doesn't ask for feedback

Doesn't care what others think

Doesn't listen

Excessively high self-appraisal

Excessively self-critical

Fears discovery of weaknesses

Not curious

Too much success

Arrogant

DEVELOPMENTAL DIFFICULTY

When compared with other dimensions of Learning Agility, this dimension is ***moderately difficult*** to develop.

🔍 Did You Know?

Experienced executive coaches report that close to 90% of leaders lack self-awareness in one or more areas. Distorted or inflated self-perception is a widespread problem. One poll found that 90% of leaders believe that they are in the top 10% of performers.[4] What's the harm in such pervasive self-esteem? It can allow blind spots to go unchecked until otherwise smart, successful leaders find their careers taking a negative turn. Blind spots are weaknesses that leaders can't see in themselves, even though they are evident to everyone around them. Research shows that blind spots are often related to low performance appraisal ratings. The three most common blind spots for executives are Making Tough People Calls, Demonstrating Personal Flexibility, and Getting Work Done Through Others.[5]

TIPS TO INCREASE SKILL IN SELF-KNOWLEDGE

Think self-reflection and self-awareness is unnecessary? Change your attitude.

RECOGNIZE THE BUSINESS BENEFITS OF KNOWING YOURSELF
Building self-awareness requires some self-reflection. You may find yourself rolling your eyes and equating self-reflection with navel-gazing and people seeking enlightenment. Self-knowledge is not some new-age fad. Self-awareness translates into positive business results. Research shows that companies that have leaders who are self-aware have higher market value and better business results. Make self-knowledge a business imperative for yourself and your team.

THINK ABOUT HOW MAKING A CHANGE COULD BENEFIT YOU
Take a hard look in the mirror. Are there recurring themes in your life that you would like to change? Whether unhelpful patterns have shown up in personal relationships or your personal ambitions, ask yourself what role have you played in these recurring themes? Then ask what is it about the trajectory of your life's story that you would like to see altered? It's hard to take control of something you are not aware of or refuse to see. Some thoughtful analysis will help you see how these patterns unfold and call a time-out before you go down the same old path.

RECOGNIZE THE DOWNSIDE OF GETTING COMFORTABLE WITH WHO YOU ARE
Even Maya Angelou, someone widely recognized as wise, recognizes that she has not arrived, that she is "in process." There is no such thing as a stationary understanding of yourself. Just when you think you have yourself figured out,

FACTOR I: SELF~AWARENESS

5

you change. Stay nimble and ready to learn new things about yourself. Let yourself evolve. Let your understanding of yourself be "in process." Focus more on the practices of self-reflection than on the illusive destination of finding 100% clarity regarding who you are.

RESOURCES TO LEARN MORE

Harvard Business Review. (2010). *HBR's 10 must reads on managing yourself.* Boston, MA: Harvard Business School Press.

Winfrey, O. (2000, December). Oprah talks to Maya Angelou [Interview]. *O, The Oprah Magazine.*

Need to learn more about yourself?
Make sense of the feedback you're getting.

ASK FOR FEEDBACK FROM PEOPLE AROUND YOU

When you get feedback, you can compare your impressions of yourself with the other people's perceptions of you. This can be enlightening. But feedback is only useful when it is honest. Make sure you're ready to listen and demonstrate that to others. Otherwise, people will be discouraged from giving you honest feedback in the future. Research shows that by genuinely seeking feedback and admitting your weaknesses to others, you actually improve their perception of you.

CHECK IN WITH THOSE AROUND YOU

People are almost as reluctant to give feedback as they are to receive it. One way to get some informal feedback is to state what you already think about your behavior and see if your hunch checks out with those around you. "I think I rushed the concluding remarks a bit, did it seem that way to you?" Or, "I'm afraid I may have alienated some folks, what do you think?" This informal, open-ended check-in can be just the invitation your colleagues, boss, or direct reports need to muster the courage to give you their point of view.

Be careful not to become overreliant on other people's feedback. If you start to check in with others before you dare make a move or a statement, then you are probably overly self-conscious. Balance concern for others' perceptions with the ability to proceed with confidence.

REFLECT ON ROOT CAUSES

Thinking about the root of the issue can be helpful in determining an action plan. Ask why: Why am I seen this way? How did my strengths get to be so? Are my weaknesses things I avoid, things I am simply not skilled at, things I dislike, or things I've never done? What experiences shaped my pattern? Do I have strengths that are related to my weaknesses, such as the smart person who makes others feel less so? Use this analysis to determine what is relatively easier and tougher for you to do.

RESOURCES TO LEARN MORE

Ingram, D. (2012). What are the benefits of 360 degree feedback? *Chron.com*

Vajda, P. (2007, December 13). Asking co-workers for feedback. *Helium*.

Scared of what you might find?
Be courageous.

FIGURE OUT WHAT IS HOLDING YOU BACK

What happens when something is amiss? Maybe you are unable to make the impact or get the results you and others expect. You may be tempted to blame the situation, find fault in others, or shrug your shoulders and leave it a mystery. But you know those are not fruitful options. On the other hand, seeking feedback about your skills and behaviors requires courage. Find the support you need. Summon the courage required to gather and analyze feedback to figure out what is holding you back from achieving your potential.

WATCH THE DEFENSIVENESS

When you do not agree that a skill deficit is as bad as others are saying, you may start to get defensive. Maybe you're in denial about a weakness or unable to accept that your weakness is really such a big problem. Stark disagreement with consistent feedback from others usually means that you do not know yourself very well. Your goal is to narrow the gap between your own and others' perceptions. Gaining additional insight and building self-awareness can help you avoid trouble. Self-aware leaders are more likely to be higher performers and have greater long-term career success.

BE WILLING TO ACKNOWLEDGE THAT YOU ARE COMPLEX

Sometimes it's hard to make sense of the feedback because it's intermittent and inconsistent. It's possible, for example, that your peers view you as compassionate, but your direct reports don't. Or your boss thinks you are a strong problem solver, but your peers think you have a weakness there. More often than not, these types of scenarios are a result of behavior on your part that is context- or situation-dependent. In fact, you may behave differently with people in the same constituency—for example, being viewed as approachable by two direct reports but not by a third. Just because the feedback is inconsistent or you don't understand the problem doesn't mean there isn't a problem. The way to move ahead in these situations is to get additional sources of credible feedback.

5

RESOURCES TO LEARN MORE

Herbold, R. J. (2011). *What's holding you back: 10 Bold steps that define gutsy leaders.* San Francisco, CA: Jossey-Bass.

Reddy, K. (2012, February 27). Now, don't get defensive, but. . . *Financial Post.*

ASSIGNMENTS TO PRACTICE SKILL

Shadow someone who is an expert at something you've never done before, go back to school, build a new skill. By formally studying something new and taking time to reflect, you are more aware of what you know and what you don't know.

Work outside of your home country and culture. Whether you relocate, manage a global team, or interview customers from different regions, use the opportunity to build awareness of your own cultural norms, values, and identity.

Make peace with an enemy or someone you've disappointed or someone you've had some trouble with or don't get along with very well. Focus on what you contributed to the situation—not what they did.

TAKE TIME TO REFLECT...

Here are some questions to reflect on as you focus on Self-Knowledge. Think about how you might answer these today and how, through using the tips in this chapter, you might achieve a better result in the future.

When was the last time you admitted to someone that you were wrong? What happened? How did you feel afterwards?

How do people respond to you? What kind of an impact would you like to have on others? Is there anything getting in the way? What could you change?

What personal insight about yourself has helped you most? How did you come to have that insight? What habits could help you have more personal insights on a regular basis?

....

Knowing yourself is the beginning of all wisdom.

Aristotle
Ancient Greek philosopher, scientist, and physician (384 BCE – 322 BCE)

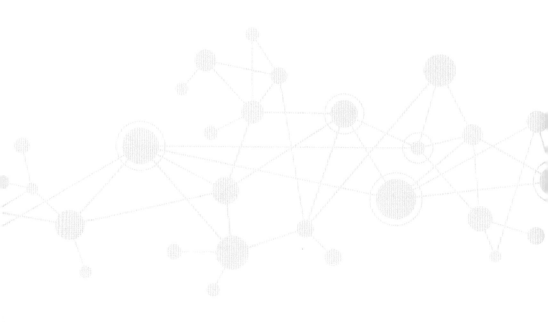

Mental Agility

While at first glance it may seem that Mental Agility is synonymous with how smart you are, that's actually not the case. It turns out that being mentally agile has much more to do with intellectual curiosity than it does with pure intellect. It's a particular kind of curiosity that drives someone with high Mental Agility. The mentally agile person is propelled by a *broad* inquisitiveness—which makes them like an intellectual explorer of the world around them. An explorer of ideas, people, history, and the future. They take in more because they are constantly scanning the environment for anything new, anything that could fuel their unquenchable desire to learn something new, to be surprised. When solving problems, this broad perspective enables the mentally agile person to make fresh connections. By accessing their bounty of broad information sources, they uncover the parallels to other things in life. Themes emerge more easily, which leads them to get at the essence or core meaning of the problem, to properly define it—the most important phase to solving anything of complexity. Someone with high Mental Agility isn't overwhelmed by complexity or ambiguity. On the contrary, the more complex or ambiguous, the greater the challenge to sift through the noisy details and distill them down into understandable themes that can be simply defined and articulated.

DIMENSIONS

Inquisitive

Broad Scanner

Connector

Essence

Complexity

Manages Uncertainty

Inquisitive

6

Inquiring, by definition, means to investigate, to question. It implies that there is some unknown waiting to be discovered, explored, and defined. Some new information, new knowledge that, once understood, will satisfy the curiosity of the seeker. But curiosity in someone who is highly inquisitive is never really satisfied. Being inquisitive means you're constantly hunting for answers to questions: What's this? How does that work? Why did that happen? What can be learned from this? Tough problems become intriguing puzzles to be solved. Learning about something new increases the chance of making novel connections when the same old solutions are falling flat. It can be tempting to default to habitual ways of thinking and acting, but sameness in this context is not your friend. If you rely solely on the familiar, your solution and idea bank will likely keep shrinking as the environment around you gets more and more complex. With a steady infusion of the fresh and new, that bank will become filled with scores of options and approaches for you to choose from.

We keep moving forward, opening new doors, and doing new things, because we're curious and curiosity keeps leading us down new paths.

Walt Disney
American film producer, director, screenwriter, and animator

SKILLED
Searches for the new

Is curious

Approaches the unknown as an adventure to be explored

Seeks new approaches to solve problems

Views mistakes as opportunities to learn

LESS SKILLED	OVERUSE OF SKILL
Likes the familiar	Focuses on unvetted ideas simply because they are new
Goes to comfortable sources	
Prefers not to challenge present conceptions	Dismisses the familiar and established without due cause
Is less at ease when things are uncertain	Explores without purpose; curiosity becomes an end unto itself, rather than a means to an end
Favors well-established solutions	
	Can't distinguish between the important and the trivial when exploring the new

SOME POSSIBLE CAUSES OF LOWER SKILL
Causes help explain "why" a person may have trouble in this dimension. When seeking to increase skill, it's helpful to consider how these might play out in certain situations. And remember that all of these can be addressed if you are motivated to do so.

Comfortable with what is	Easily frustrated
Impatient	Not curious
Intimidated by things and people who are different	Values convention
Narrow background	Confident in his/her knowledge
	Arrogant

DEVELOPMENTAL DIFFICULTY
When compared with other dimensions of Learning Agility, this dimension is **easier** to develop.

⭐ Does It Best

Among renowned physicist Albert Einstein's abundance of mental attributes, one that stands apart was his unceasing quest for new knowledge about the world around him. Einstein described it this way: "I am not more gifted than anybody else. I am just more curious than the average person, and I will not give up on a problem until I have found the proper solution."[6] Einstein's curiosity took shape well beyond the boundaries of science with philosophy, religion, politics, and music being just some of the areas he explored in his lifetime.

TIPS TO INCREASE SKILL IN BEING INQUISITIVE

Comfortable with current boundaries?
Push the limits of your comfort zone.

MAKE THE UNFAMILIAR FAMILIAR

Stimulate your brain by doing things, going places, and talking to people outside of your routine. Take a course in an area you know nothing about. Or take a course in an area only sort of related to what you do. Go to the theater, concerts, and other cultures' festivals. Vacation at places you've never been before and without doing a lot of pre-trip research. Go to restaurants you know nothing about. Attend perspective-broadening lectures and workshops on topics that you normally don't attend. Talk to more strangers in line at the grocery store and on airplanes. Change up day-to-day things—drive to work a different way, use the computer mouse with your opposite hand, rearrange your furniture. Constantly ask yourself is there anything new to learn here? Anything that may surprise me?

EXPAND YOUR TASK REPERTOIRE

Doing the same things in the same ways makes for easy thinking. But if you gravitate toward the same tasks and ways of doing things again and again, you're not leaving much room to try anything new. So if most of the tasks you do each day feel as comfortable as an old shirt, it's probably time to expand and diversify your task wardrobe. Start by making a list of what you like to do or is familiar, and what you don't like to do or is new. Do at least a couple of your liked activities each day, but not until you've tackled the don't likes or unfamiliar activities first. By pushing through and doing the tasks that are harder, require more focus, or force you to face your own ignorance on a topic, you're more likely to learn something new.

 Expanding the range of what you do is not the same as abandoning established ways of doing things without due cause. Established methods are established for a reason—they've been tested and proven over time. Find the rightful place for your tried-and-true tasks and methods.

EXTEND THE BOUNDARIES FOR "WHAT IS"

Much research from anthropology has shown that our brains are trapped inside our belief framework, which dictates how we interpret and interact with the world around us. The Hopi Indians in the southwestern United States have one word for snow. The Inuit of Alaska, on the other hand, have many different words for snow which reflect the many different ways their lives are impacted by snow and snow conditions. A Hopi could not survive in Alaska with just one snow concept. Our own experience unknowingly creates boundaries for our thinking. Try to think outside your belief boundaries. You don't have to give them up; just turn them off when you are thinking about a problem or challenge. Or, better yet, when exploring something new, compare and contrast your current framework related to that new something with the new data that you uncover.

6

RESOURCES TO LEARN MORE

Cummings, I. (2008). *The vigorous mind: Cross-train your brain to break through mental, emotional, and professional boundaries.* Deerfield Beach, FL: Health Communications, Inc.

Rubin, G. (2009, November 12). *The happiness of doing something new: The audiobook version.* The Happiness Project.

Think you have to know it all?
Make uncertainty work for you.

EMBRACE AMBIGUITY

Do you feel best when you know everything that's going on around you and you are in control? Most do. Few are motivated by uncertainty and chaos. Humans are hardwired to crave certainty. Brain research shows that we are more averse to ambiguity than risk. Why? In risk situations, the brain can weigh the pros and cons, it has something constructive to do. When things are uncertain, there is nothing to calculate, so the brain works overtime to try and decrease the uncertainty. Inquisitive people have figured out that the reward for exploring the new is worth the ambiguity that comes with it. Envision the payoff of the unknown and you'll become more comfortable being a pioneer—solving problems no one has solved before and cutting paths where no one has been before.

BE A QUESTIONER
Questions are a powerful tool—both for exploring the new and reducing uncertainty when solving problems. But as powerful as questions can be, they are often underused. In one study of problem solving, 7% of comments were questions and about half were solutions. Focusing on solutions may be efficient in the short-term but could leave you optionless if you don't deposit fresh ideas and approaches into the mix. Questions are the fuel for new ideas and new ways for solving problems. So start and keep asking why. For problems needing to be solved, asking why helps you see what the causes are so you can start to put them into organizing buckets. This increases the chance of a better solution because you can see more connections. For new ideas or ambiguous situations, asking why and how helps you uncover new insights and information for your idea engine.

GO OUT ON A LIMB
The path to learn, to explore something unknown, often involves taking a risk. The greater the unknown, the greater the risk. You can't learn anything if you're not trying anything new. The Wright brothers were determined to satisfy their curiosity about the feasibility of human flight, despite the fact that all previous attempts to fly had been failures. Research indicates that more successful people have made more mistakes than the less successful. When you're seeking to find answers to something, go for small wins so you can recover quickly if you miss, and more importantly, learn from the results. Don't try to satisfy your curiosity and expect to get it right the first time. Many problem-solving studies show that the second or third try is when we really understand the underlying dynamics of problems. Think of exploring as a series of try-learn-try again-learn some more.

RESOURCES TO LEARN MORE
Marquardt, M. J. (2005). *Leading with questions: How leaders find the right solutions by knowing what to ask.* San Francisco, CA: Jossey-Bass.
Reilly, J. M. (2012, April 18). Embracing failure on the path to success. *Entrepreneur.*

Need some techniques to get started?
Put inquisitiveness to work.

PRIME THE CURIOSITY PUMP
To fuel curiosity, it helps to think creatively. Creative thought processes do not follow the formal rules of logic—where one uses cause and effect to prove or solve something. Being creative means looking everywhere and every which way. Some rules of creative thought are:

- Move from one concept or way of looking at things to another, such as from economic to political.

- Generate ideas without judging them initially.

- Use information to restructure and come up with new patterns.

- Jump from one idea to another without justifying the jump.

- Look for parallels far from the problem, such as how is an organization like a big oak tree?

- Look for the least likely and odd.

- Ask what's missing or what's not here.

 Stay grounded and purposeful. You don't want to cultivate a reputation of being a scatterbrain. Applied curiosity may involve being impractical at first, but always to achieve very practical and useful ends.

FIND THE EXCEPTIONS AND THE OUTLIERS

Getting fresh ideas doesn't happen through quick scanning; it requires looking deeply. Carve out dedicated time—study it deeply, look for parallels in other organizations and in remote areas totally outside your field. Practice picking out anomalies—unusual facts that don't quite fit, like sales going down when they should have gone up. What do these odd things imply for strategy? Or look for distant parallels. Don't fall into the mental trap of searching only in parallel organizations to your own because "only they would know." Back up and ask a broader question to aid in the search for solutions. When Motorola wanted to find out how to process orders more quickly, they went not to other electronics firms, but to Domino's Pizza and FedEx. If your response to this is that you don't have the time, that also usually explains why you're not having any fresh ideas.

FRESHEN TRADITIONAL PROBLEM SOLVING

When confronted with a new, fresh problem, it's helpful to take a fresh approach to solving it. So turn the problem upside down: ask what is the least likely thing it could be, what the problem is not, what's missing from the problem, or what the mirror image of the problem is. Sometimes going to extremes helps. Exploring every condition, every worst case you can think of sometimes will suggest a different solution. Taking the present state of affairs and projecting into the future may indicate how and where the system will break down. It also helps to think out loud. Many people don't know what they know until they talk it out. Find a good sounding board and talk to him/her to increase your understanding of a problem or a technical area. Talk to an expert in an unrelated field. Talk to the most irreverent person you know. Your goal is not to get their input but, rather, help in figuring out what *you* know (and don't know).

RESOURCES TO LEARN MORE

Blakely, D. (2011, March 14). Fostering innovation [Video file]. Stanford Graduate School of Business.

Sternberg, R. J. (2007). *Wisdom, intelligence, and creativity synthesized*. New York, NY: Cambridge University Press.

ASSIGNMENTS TO PRACTICE SKILL

Start something from scratch that will require doing a lot of first-time things and meeting new challenges that might need fixing in a short period of time.

Take on a role much bigger than the one you have now. The larger scope and complexity will mean managing a high variety of activities at different levels of complexity and certainty.

Go global with an international assignment that will involve thinking through tough problems from a novel position and for this new setting, which will likely be different from your own background.

TAKE TIME TO REFLECT...

Here are some questions to reflect on as you focus on being Inquisitive. Think about how you might answer these today and how, through using the tips in this chapter, you might achieve a better result in the future.

Remember back to your childhood and that wonderful feeling of uncovering the secret to something you didn't know before. How can you capture that sense of discovery, of newness, in the world around you? How can you think like a child today?

Capture three things you would like to explore in more detail— additional questions to pose, research to gather, etc. When will you start pursuing these efforts? What will your plan be?

Identify one current situation that would benefit from additional questions or inquiry. What information is needed? What answers would prove valuable to shaping the situation or outcome? Where can you flex your inquisitive muscle?

Count how many times you've returned to the same restaurant, vacation spot, leisure activity. How much does it take for you to try something new, something that is truly foreign or unfamiliar to you? What do you have to lose?

....

People say: idle curiosity.
The one thing that curiosity cannot be is idle.

Leo Rosten
Polish-American author and humorist

7

Broad
Scanner

When you're around a Broad Scanner, you're likely to hear them describe something as "fascinating." Broad Scanners find something inherently fascinating in just about everything—in people, in ideas, in history, in the future, in the world at large. They explore a variety of diverse sources, making it possible to extract insights that would otherwise be elusive. It's like viewing the world around you in wide-screen—you take in more and gain more resources to draw upon. Ideas, perspectives, and strategies come more from a prepared mind than from raw intelligence or creativity. They come from a mind broadened by lots of varied but disconnected experiences, exposures, and interests. As you tackle new ideas, complex problems, and first-time situations, this kind of broad outlook will give you a greater repertoire to draw from and more chances to come up with meaningful connections in your life and work.

A man practices the art of adventure when he breaks the chain of routine and renews his life through reading new books, traveling to new places, making new friends, taking up new hobbies and adopting new viewpoints.

Wilfred Peterson
American author and newspaper columnist

SKILLED

Knowledgeable on a range of work and non-work topics

Uses multiple lenses to view problems and opportunities

Calls upon a wide variety of sources in brainstorming activities

Gets involved with a lot of different things

Uses examples from history and biography to find common themes across different topics

Reads broadly

LESS SKILLED

May use limited sources or media for knowledge

Relies on personal experience when solving problems

Doesn't have far-ranging interests

Views situations from his/her own unique point of view

Can only find commonalities when topics are closely related

OVERUSE OF SKILL

Gets fixated on every trivial piece of information

Becomes a font of useless information without any productive purpose

Can be seen as a know-it-all

More interested in demonstrating own knowledge than solving problems

Brings so many sources into the mix that own opinion gets lost

SOME POSSIBLE CAUSES OF LOWER SKILL

Causes help explain "why" a person may have trouble in this dimension. When seeking to increase skill, it's helpful to consider how these might play out in certain situations. And remember that all of these can be addressed if you are motivated to do so.

Too busy

Doesn't value information not needed now

Impatient

Low curiosity

Narrow band of friends, acquaintances

Prefers depth to broad

Highly specialized

Limited experience

One-dimensional thinker

Values only practical knowledge

DEVELOPMENTAL DIFFICULTY

When compared with other dimensions of Learning Agility, this dimension is **_easier_** to develop.

🔆 Did You Know?

As the world becomes more interconnected and complex, having a broad perspective has become more important to performance at the manager and executive levels, according to recent research. Further, in one of the most comprehensive studies that followed the careers of successful employees for 35 years, researchers found that one of the best predictors of success was a range of interests.

TIPS TO INCREASE SKILL AS A BROAD SCANNER

Married to favorite information sources?
Broaden your information horizon.

STUDY THE MASTERS

Select a biography of a historical figure you admire but don't know much about. What made the figure significant? What were his/her key accomplishments and contributions? What were critical lessons in his/her life? Write down five things you can emulate in your own behavior. Beyond historical figures, you can study a few great thinkers and philosophers like John Stuart Mill who outlined the basic logic of problem solving. Read their biographies or autobiographies for clues into how they used their intellectual skills.

READ WIDELY

Read publications with global reach and coverage like *Commentary*, the *Economist, Monocle*, or the *International Herald Tribune*. Check out "we present all sides" journals like the *Atlantic* to get the broadest possible view of issues. Read an autobiography of someone with global insights like Henry Kissinger. Pick a country and study it. Or think about world events through the perspectives of other cultures. What's the Russian view of the Middle East? What drives the French economy? How does Turkey control the water supply to many countries? You're likely to find common underlying principles that you can apply to what you're doing today.

CHANNEL YOUR INNER INNOVATOR

Become a student of innovation outside your field. Look for and study new products you buy and use. Find out the process that was used to create it. Watch the History Channel's *Modern Marvels*. Read Pulitzer Prize winning *The Soul of a New Machine* by Tracy Kidder to see how innovation happens from the inside. See how innovators use the past to predict the future. How several unrelated inventions came together to form a bigger one. Write down five things from your research that you can model in your own behavior, then put them into practice.

The more diverse sources of information you use, the greater the temptation to call them up as evidence to support your position on something. If you're not careful, you may end up sounding like an encyclopedia. It's important to acquire a broad perspective, but be sure not to lose your own.

RESOURCES TO LEARN MORE

Berkun, S. (2010). *The myths of innovation*. Sebastopol, CA: O'Reilly Media, Inc.

Biography Channel. biography.com

Focused only on your immediate work?
Broaden your understanding of the business.

LEARN THE SPECIFICS OF YOUR BUSINESS

On your own, study your organization's annual report and various financial reports. If you don't know how, the major investment firms have basic documents explaining how to read financials. Once you've studied up, consult a pro and ask what they look at and why. Reach out to the person in charge of the strategic planning process in your company. Have them explain the strategic plan—how is the organization addressing external market forces like globalization, changing demographics, world financial uncertainties? Does your firm differentiate through customer intimacy, innovation, operational excellence? Particularly, have them point out the mission-critical functions and capabilities the organization needs to be on the leading edge in order to win. Be a sponge for knowledge about your business, your customers, and your competitors.

GET A MEDIA DOWNLOAD ON THE BUSINESS LANDSCAPE OF TODAY AND TOMORROW

Read the *Wall Street Journal* and *Bloomberg Businessweek* and write down three to five interesting things that have a parallel or an effect on your organization. Learn to connect what's out there to what's in here. Start reading periodicals such as the *New Yorker, Forbes, Fortune,* and *Bloomberg Businessweek*. Keep a log of ideas you get from each. Want a crystal ball into future business concerns? Read any of the *Megatrends* books by John Naisbitt, the *Popcorn Report* by Faith Popcorn, or the *Futurist*, a journal of the World Future Society. These publications and others like them raise issues such as what does it mean that the birth rate is collapsing in the developed world? By 2030, it is estimated that half of Japan's population will be 65 or older. Much the same is true in the rest of the developed world. Will the retirement age go up? Leisure spending may go down since more time off is not likely. Education and health care professionals will grow. Second and third "careers" will be standard. The means of production has largely become knowledge. Outsourcing is up—knowledge is increasingly specialized, expensive, and difficult to maintain. Is this a harbinger of more outsourcing and alliances? Or, as knowledge jobs become commoditized, will there be a premium on ideas, on design, on what Daniel Pink calls "high concept and high touch" abilities? What are the trends at play and how do they affect your organization going forward?

APPRENTICE YOURSELF

Find an expert or experts in your functional/technical/business area and go find out how they think and solve new problems. Ask them what critical principles/drivers/things they look for in their work. Have them tell you how they thought through a new problem in this area, the major skills they look for in sizing up people's proficiency in this area, key questions they ask about a problem, how they would suggest you go about learning quickly in this area. Most don't mind having a few "apprentices" around, so ask whether they would mind showing you the ropes and tutoring you. Ask, "How do you know what's important? What do you look at first? Second? What are the five keys you always look at or for? What do you read? Who do you go to for advice?"

RESOURCES TO LEARN MORE

Fast Company. fastcompany.com

Pink, D. (2005). *A whole new mind: Why right-brainers will rule the future.* New York, NY: Penguin Books.

Learn by doing?
Broaden your experiences.

BROADEN YOUR WORK ROUTINE

Maybe you haven't seen enough in your current and past roles. Pick some activities you haven't done before but might find exciting and challenging. Take advantage of training events or knowledge-sharing opportunities your company offers. Task trade with a peer. Volunteer for task forces and projects that are multifunctional or multibusiness in nature. To broaden your outlook, multi or different are the key words to look for in seeking these kinds of opportunities.

EXPLORE THINGS WELL OUT OF YOUR NORM

A key reason we humans so readily stick to routines and the familiar is because research shows our brains are set up to like it that way. To override the brain's laziness, study and dabble in three unrelated things that you have not paid much attention to before—opera, romance novels, technical journals out of your area, MTV, learn a new language, take a magic course, study archeology. How do the principles of one tie into the other? Ask yourself what common truths or insights you can gain about human nature, the way things work, and about yourself.

 Use your knowledge only for good. While it may be tempting to gush about all you know on a wide range of topics, you may end up coming across as arrogant or patronizing to those around you. Save your "for instances" and "did you knows" for times when they will add value to problem solving and idea generation.

EXPERIENCE PEOPLE NOT JUST LIKE YOU

Spend time socially or at work functions (lunches, outings) with those who are broad in viewpoint and diverse in background. Pay attention to topics they discuss that you aren't versed in. Make a point to learn or discover new information from them. Consider researching or investigating those topics afterward to learn more so that you can converse with them at the next encounter. Find opportunities to assemble a team of people of varying perspectives and backgrounds. Studies show that teams of people with the widest diversity of backgrounds produce the most innovative solutions to problems. Get others with different backgrounds to analyze and make sense of issues with you.

RESOURCES TO LEARN MORE

Duhigg, C. (2012). *The power of habit: Why we do what we do in life and business.* New York, NY: Random House, Inc.

Porter, M. E. (2008). *On competition.* Boston, MA: Harvard Business School Press.

ASSIGNMENTS TO PRACTICE SKILL

Move to a different function or business unit or region where you will start off as a novice and only be successful by acquiring a broadened understanding.

Assemble a team of diverse people to accomplish a difficult task. Use the opportunity to both get the job done and build up your people-differences perspective.

Study a new trend, product, service, technique, or process you have never experienced before.

TAKE TIME TO REFLECT...

Here are some questions to reflect on as you focus on being a Broad Scanner. Think about how you might answer these today and how, through using the tips in this chapter, you might achieve a better result in the future.

How can you make space in an already crowded life to expand your horizons? In what ways can you pair learning about new things with getting things done?

What are you interested in learning more about? What processes are in place that you have always wondered why or how they work? Where could you benefit from different functional perspectives?

How has a new experience, product, or concept shaped your views? How has this helped broaden your perspectives? How is your thinking different today?

Where might a fresh perspective benefit you? Where might you be stalling or blinded because of your own frame of reference? What will you do to ensure you incorporate fresh perspectives into important decisions?

The more that you read, the more things you will know.
The more that you learn, the more places you'll go.

Dr. Seuss
American author and artist

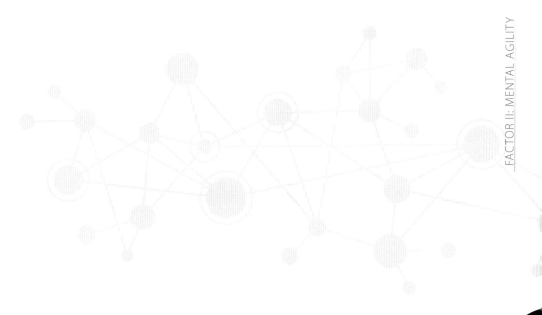

Connector

8

Creative problem solving starts with making creative connections. Connections uncovered by finding commonality between two or more unrelated knowns. If you restrict yourself to the connections you currently make, you'll only come up with breakthrough ideas by sheer chance. Or you may end up faced with a situation where there is no obvious connection to lean on. Being a Connector enables you to see beyond the obvious. To look underneath the surface features of an issue, problem, or set of conditions to find the in-common, the patterns, in what seems to be completely unrelated but isn't. Similar things happen in parallel areas of life. Almost nothing is truly new. Almost everything has already happened. Spotting trends isn't going to happen by being myopic and only looking insular to your own experience. You can increase your chances of success by learning from the lessons of history and making connections across usually isolated areas. Research of star performers from global companies like Volvo and IBM revealed that the one cognitive ability that distinguished them from average performers was pattern recognition, which allowed them to pick out meaningful trends and use that information to solve future problems.

In nature we never see anything isolated,
but everything in connection with something else
which is before it, beside it, under it and over it.

Johann Wolfgang von Goethe
German playwright, poet, novelist, and dramatist

SKILLED

Combines two or more disparate ideas to create something new

Finds parallels, contrasts, and unique combinations

Isn't afraid to go off on an intellectual tangent and take time to think through something

Comes up with missing pieces

Finds commonality among seemingly contrasting data

Identifies patterns in seemingly unrelated pieces of information

LESS SKILLED

Focuses on what is readily apparent

May think he/she already knows the answer

Too quick to act

Doesn't hunt for fresh views or solutions

Sees little value in looking for seemingly obscure parallels

OVERUSE OF SKILL

Doggedly insists that patterns or themes exist, even when all evidence is to the contrary

Gets so caught up in connection-finding that deadlines are missed

Rejects the obvious solution without due consideration

SOME POSSIBLE CAUSES OF LOWER SKILL

Causes help explain "why" a person may have trouble in this dimension. When seeking to increase skill, it's helpful to consider how these might play out in certain situations. And remember that all of these can be addressed if you are motivated to do so.

Impatient

Intellectually lazy

Limited ways to think

Narrow or disadvantaged background

Not curious

Rejects speculation

Sticks with the proven

Too specialized

Rigid mental models

Overly focused

Unobservant

DEVELOPMENTAL DIFFICULTY

When compared with other dimensions of Learning Agility, this dimension is **moderately difficult** to develop.

Did You Know?

A 2003 research study commissioned for the British Broadcasting Company found that self-made millionaires are four times more likely than the rest of us to be dyslexic.[7] The connection to being a Connector? While a person with dyslexia has difficulty analyzing particulars, they are very adept at recognizing patterns.[8]

TIPS TO INCREASE SKILL AS A CONNECTOR

Only seeing the obvious?
Be unconventional.

REMOVE THE RESTRAINTS

Many busy people rely too much on solutions from their own history. They rely on what has happened to them in the past. They see sameness in problems that isn't there. Beware of "I have always…" or "Usually, I…." Always pause and ask yourself is this really like the problems you have solved in the past? You don't have to change who you are and what you're comfortable with other than when you need to be more creative in your thinking. First think, then act, differently; try new things; break free of your restraints.

MAKE YOUR MIND A BIT SILLIER

If you're driven by logic, you may be limiting your ability to make fresh connections. Don't be afraid to think illogically for a change. You don't have to tell anyone what you're doing. Think about what song this problem is like. Find an analogy to your problem in nature, in children's toys, in anything that has a physical structure. Engineers once solved an overheating problem by drawing a parallel to what animal trainers do to calm upset or angry animals. Seemingly silly parallels can reveal unique connections.

TAP INTO NON-EXPERTS

During World War II, the military discovered the most creative groups were those where the members had little or nothing in common and knew little about the issue. Their freewheeling approach yielded fresher solutions. They were not trapped by the past. Experts in strategic planning often use this tactic today to ensure they are bringing in the broadest way to look at how future scenarios may take shape. Take a current challenge to the most disparate group you can find (a historian, a college student, a theologian, a salesperson, a plumber, etc.) and see what insights they have into it. Find some problems outside of *your* area and see what you can add.

RESOURCES TO LEARN MORE

Day, P. (2009, June 23). Mind of a millionaire. BBC series.

Shaughnessy, H. (2011, June 24). The new work manifesto: Be unconventional. *Forbes*.

Too focused on a solution?
Think it through.

AVOID A QUICK MOVE TO SOLUTIONING

One reason people jump to solutions based on what has worked in the past is impatience. Life is a balance between waiting and doing. Many in management put a premium on doing over waiting. Most of us could make close to 100% good decisions, given all of the data and unlimited time. Life affords us neither the data nor the time. Try to discipline yourself to wait just a little longer than you usually do to come up with a solution. Push yourself to always look at one more piece of data than you did before. You'll find that what you sacrifice in speed, you gain in quality of the solution.

 Ensuring you have a good understanding of a problem before solving preemptively is certainly a good thing, but slowing down to a snail's pace is not. When tackling problems and ideas creatively, be sure to balance thorough analysis with a bias for action.

DEFINE THE PROBLEM

Fresh connections don't occur in a vacuum. You need information so you have something to go on. When solving problems, start with figuring out what causes it in the first place. See how many causes you can come up with and how many organizing buckets you can put them in. Many of us just collect data, which numerous studies show increases our confidence but doesn't increase decision accuracy. Think out loud with others, see how they view the problem. Studies show that defining the problem and taking action usually occur simultaneously, so to break out of analysis paralysis, figure out what the problem is first. Then, when a good alternative appears, you're likely to recognize it immediately.

TAKE TIME TO ASK QUESTIONS

Instead of just doing it, ask what questions would need to be answered before we'd know which way to go. Too often, we think first and only of solutions. In studies of problem-solving sessions, solutions outweigh questions eight to one. When thinking through problems creatively with others, it's typical for the meeting to start with people offering solutions. Often, others haven't even understood the problem yet! Plus, early solutions are not likely to be the best. So set aside the first 50% of the time for questions and problem definition and the last 50% of the time for solutions. Asking more questions early helps you rethink the problem and come to more and different solutions.

RESOURCES TO LEARN MORE

Cashman, K. (2012). The pause principle: *Step back to lead forward.* San Francisco, CA: Berrett-Koehler Publishers, Inc.

The Systems Thinker®. Waltham, MA: Pegasus Communications, Inc. 781-398-9700. www.thesystemsthinker.com

Trouble connecting the dots?
Start seeing the patterns in things.

EXPLORE THE IN-COMMONS

Look for patterns and commonalities across seemingly unrelated stories, events, or circumstances. The broader your outlook, the more patterns you are likely to see. Look for patterns everywhere: in your personal life, your organization, or the world when analyzing general successes and failures. What was common to each success or what was present in each failure but never present in a success? Focus more on the successes; failures are easier to analyze but don't in themselves tell you what *would* have worked. Comparing successes, while less exciting, yields more information about underlying principles. The bottom line is to reduce your insights to principles or rules of thumb you think might be repeatable. When faced with the next new problem, those general underlying principles will apply again.

HUNT FOR REMOTE PARALLELS

Parallels exist everywhere—in your own business, in other organizations, and in remote areas totally outside your field. Parallels aren't necessarily best practices, which come and go. Instead, find a parallel situation to the underlying issue you are solving—like who has to do things really fast (Domino's Pizza, FedEx)? Who has to deal with maximum ambiguity (emergency rooms, a newspaper, police dispatchers)? Achievements in innovation can be another great source for parallels. Study a few well-known inventions of the past, like the automobile (*The Machine That Changed the World* by James Womack and associates at MIT is an excellent source). See how several unrelated inventions came together to form a bigger one.

USE HISTORY AS A GUIDE

If you feel stuck in the present, start seeing what patterns emerge from history. There are always plenty of candidates. U.S. president Harry Truman used the presidential archives to form a "council of presidents" to see what his predecessors had done in parallel situations to the issues he was facing. Studying the biographies of three creative people without regard to their field can be a great source of inspiration as well. See what processes they shared in common that helped them be more creative in their thinking and what kinds of unique connections they were able to make as a result.

 Once you begin seeing the power of making new connections, it can be tempting to expect to find them in every situation. It's important to keep in mind that overcomplicating a topic for the sake of hunting for connections and patterns needs to have a payoff attached. And that sometimes the obvious solution is the best one.

RESOURCES TO LEARN MORE

Grothe, M. (2008). *I never metaphor I didn't like: A comprehensive compilation of history's greatest analogies, metaphors, and similes.* New York, NY: Harper Collins.

Levi, S. (2004). *Use history like a tool: An unconventional guide to reading the past and managing the future.* Aberdeen, WA: Silver Lake Publishing.

ASSIGNMENTS TO PRACTICE SKILL

Work in a strategic planning role or on a cross-functional project that will provide you with lots of fodder to make fresh connections, analyze multiple new ideas, and devise new ways of looking at old problems.

Start something new. To be successful, you'll need to find parallels between your new venture or situation and examples from the world around you and then make connections that will help you forge ahead.

Work on a team tasked with fixing something that has failed. You can bring in lessons about others' failures and successes, connect the in-commons with your situation, and use that knowledge to strategize how to solve what needs fixing.

TAKE TIME TO REFLECT...

Here are some questions to reflect on as you focus on being a Connector. Think about how you might answer these today and how, through using the tips in this chapter, you might achieve a better result in the future.

Think about people or companies you admire. What is it that draws you to them? What do they all have in common?

How often do you have your solution already in mind before any real exploration of a new problem has begun? What is the impact?

When was the last time you made a connection that was so exciting it gave you goose bumps?

....

Discovery consists of seeing what everybody has seen
and thinking what nobody has thought.

Albert Szent-Gyorgyi
Hungarian physiologist and winner of the Nobel Prize in medicine

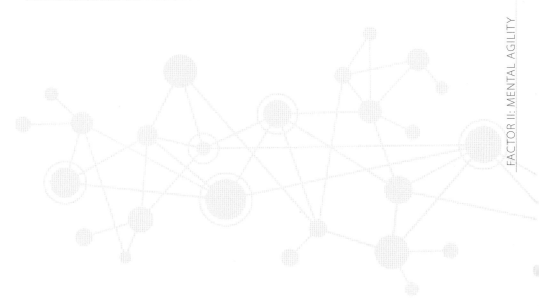

∞

91

Essence

9

To uncover the meaning, the essence, of a problem, issue, or challenge often starts with asking *why*—why is this a problem? Or asking *how*—how is this problem like others? It can be tempting to just focus on the surface features, or the *what* of a problem, issue, or challenge. After all, the what is usually most evident and easiest to identify. But being able to describe the surface features of a problem will only get you so far. Skimming the surface often leads to superficial solutions, temporary fixes, Band-Aids that may seem appealing in the short-term but don't get at the core of what's broken. Getting to the essence of something is more like a marathon than a sprint. Those "aha" moments that may seem to happen spontaneously are usually the result of careful study. Of peeling back the layers of the problem and using connections from like or unlike examples to confirm that, yes, this is the reason why! By looking to patterns and causes of how and why something works (or doesn't work), you can produce a more robust solution and gain insights to help solve future problems.

There is more going on beneath the surface than we think, and more going on in little, finite moments of time than we would guess.

Malcolm Gladwell

British-Canadian journalist, bestselling author, speaker, and *New Yorker* columnist

SKILLED

Extracts the core meaning out of complex situations

Is able to separate the important from the noise when problem solving

Searches for the meaning behind outcomes

Investigates why and how projects were successful

Looks for themes within and across situations

Hunts for the root cause of successes and failures

LESS SKILLED

Focuses more on the *what* of a problem and less on understanding *why* and *how*

Considers only current conditions when evaluating problems

Has outsized bias for action

Struggles with problems where there isn't one clear solution or outcome

Has difficulty differentiating the various elements of a problem

Satisfied with temporary fixes to tough problems

OVERUSE OF SKILL

Force fits themes where reasonable evidence suggests there are none

May wait too long to come to a conclusion

May overcomplicate things

SOME POSSIBLE CAUSES OF LOWER SKILL

Causes help explain "why" a person may have trouble in this dimension. When seeking to increase skill, it's helpful to consider how these might play out in certain situations. And remember that all of these can be addressed if you are motivated to do so.

Doesn't go deep

High need for speed

High need to close

Impatient

Not curious

Tactically oriented

Oversimplifies

DEVELOPMENTAL DIFFICULTY

When compared with other dimensions of Learning Agility, this dimension is ***moderately difficult*** to develop.

⭐ Does It Best

Malcolm Gladwell, best-selling author and prolific *New Yorker* columnist, has made a career out of looking at problems from different angles and distilling something complex, with multiple moving parts, down to its essence. Gladwell is never satisfied with the surface explanation for a problem or situation. His topics cover a wide range: from surfacing the fundamental flaw that doomed a multinational corporation, to naming what's really behind individual success, to explaining why flavored varieties of ketchup will never sell.[9] Gladwell's counterintuitive approach challenges conventional wisdom in the spirit of uncovering the true meaning behind complex problems. His keen insights have relevance not just to business but to life in general.

TIPS TO INCREASE SKILL IN ESSENCE

Focus more on getting to solutions?
Make understanding the problem the goal.

KEEP IMPATIENCE AT BAY

Many of us are very action oriented. It's the famous fire-ready-aim. Many mistakes we make would not have happened if we had taken the time to think things through. Impatient people provide answers, conclusions, and solutions too early in the process. Brainstorm what questions need to be answered in order to resolve it. When brainstorming with others, give them the task to think about it for a day and come back with some solutions. Be a teacher instead of a dictator of solutions. Brain research shows that breakthrough insights come from our subconscious, from our "out of awareness" brain. So be patient. Take a pause before rushing to a solution.

CHECK FOR COMMON ERRORS IN THINKING

If you find you're often missing the point when tackling complex issues, it's helpful to think about how you typically approach them. Do you state as facts things that are really opinions or assumptions? Do your feelings or emotions get in the way of issues? Do you attribute cause and effect to relationships when you don't know if one causes the other? Do you generalize from a single example? Do you treat all aspects of a problem as if they are equally important? To get to the essence of something, it's important to be able to distinguish the important elements from the noisy details that don't help get to the best solution.

DEFINE THE PROBLEM

Studies show that defining the problem and taking action occur almost simultaneously for most people, so the more effort you put on the front end, the easier it is to come up with a good solution. So stop and first define what the problem is and isn't. For one-half of the time you have to deal with an issue or a problem, shut off your solution machine and just take in the facts. Since providing solutions is so easy for everyone, it would be nice if they were offering solutions to the right problem.

RESOURCES TO LEARN MORE

Finkelstein, S., Whitehead, J., & Campbell, A. (2009). *Think again: Why good leaders make bad decisions and how to keep it from happening to you.* Boston, MA: Harvard Business School Press.

Grohol, J. M. (2012). 15 Common cognitive distortions. *Psych Central*.

Unsure how to tackle tough problems?
View the problem with fresh eyes.

TURN OFF YOUR DEFAULT SOLUTION SWITCH

When you're faced with a new or tough problem or issue that needs solving, pause before defaulting to what's been the tried-and-true path for you in the past. If the solution or course of action feels comfortable—that's a red flag. If it seems like a winner on the surface—another red flag. Remember that your favored solutions likely have a shelf life. You are bound to encounter new contexts. Different people. Unfamiliar problems. Instead of defaulting, go through a mental checklist to see if you have thought about all of the ramifications of the problem or challenge. Research has shown that the first thing or solution you think of is seldom the best choice. Usually somewhere between the second and third choice turns out to be the most effective.

STUDY SUCCESSES AND ASK WHAT THEY HAVE IN COMMON

If you can find three times that something worked, ask why it worked despite differences in the situations. What was common to each success or what was present in each failure but never present in a success? Focus more on the successes; comparing successes, while less exciting, yields more information about underlying principles. Then you are on the way to finding principles that may repeat. Look for personal patterns, organizational patterns, or world patterns. The bottom line is to reduce your insights to principles or rules of thumb you think might be repeatable. When faced with the next new problem, those general underlying principles will apply again.

SEARCH FOR ESSENCE FROM UNLIKELY SOURCES

Hunt for parallels in other organizations and in remote areas totally outside your field. By this, we don't mean best practices, which come and go. Find a parallel situation to the underlying issue—for example, who has to manage to razor-thin profit margins (grocery stores, airlines)? Access a broad range of resources to find commonalities. Look beyond what's in close proximity. Ask what in nature parallels your problem. When the terrible surfs and motion of the tide threatened to defeat their massive dam project known as the Delta Works, the Dutch used the violence of the North Sea to drive in the pilings, ending the danger of the southern Netherlands flooding.

RESOURCES TO LEARN MORE

Gigerenzer, G. (2007). *Gut feelings: The intelligence of the unconscious.* New York, NY: Penguin Group.

Gladwell, M. (2007). *Blink: The power of thinking without thinking.* New York, NY: Little, Brown and Company.

**Ready to decode the problem?
Get to the core of it.**

UNCOVER KEY ELEMENTS

What are the key factors or characteristics in this problem? Experts usually solve problems by figuring out what the deep underlying principles are and working forward from there; the less adept focus on desired outcomes/ solutions and either work backward or concentrate on the surface facts. See how many causes you can come up with and how many categories you can put them in. Then ask what they have in common and how they are different. This increases the chance of a more creative solution because you can see more connections. Be a chess master. Chess masters recognize thousands of patterns of chess pieces. Look for patterns in data, don't just collect information. Put it in categories that make sense to you. Ask lots of questions. Allot at least 50% of the time to defining the problem.

DIG FOR ROOT CAUSES

Keep asking why. LEAN manufacturing, Six Sigma, and companies like Toyota use the "5 Whys" approach for root cause analysis. First, describe the problem statement. Then, ask, Why does this occur? Why does this problem exist? After the first answer, ask Why again for a total of five times. Here's an example of a problem around employee engagement:

Problem Statement: Employees are unhappy because they don't feel supported in developing their careers.

- Why? Because they are bored by working in one area, discipline, practice.

- Why? Because their development needs are not being considered, either in staffing assignments or in job rotations.
- Why? Because senior leaders prefer individuals they know and who have demonstrated skills/experiences.
- Why? Because they don't have visibility to other talent.
- Why? Because there is no regular staffing/talent management mechanism in place that is informed by individual development needs.

 Properly balance the rigor of your analysis with the speed needed to resolve an issue or challenge. You don't want the "why" asked to be, "Why are we belaboring this exercise?"

FIND THE SIMPLEST (BUT NOT SIMPLISTIC) SOLUTION FOR A PROBLEM

When a problem is complex, it may seem like a complex solution is the only way to solve it. Yet for centuries of the history of thought, the proposition has been put forward that the solution with the least number of elements or factors is probably the most correct one. Often referred to as *Ockham's razor*, or the law of economy or parsimony, the principle is that if there are two or more equally valid ways to explain something, it's best to proceed with the simplest. See how few reasons you can create that explain the issue. When it comes time to follow through on the solution, you'll have something simpler, more explainable, and repeatable to work with.

> **RESOURCES TO LEARN MORE**
> Andersen, B., & Fagerhaug, T. (2006). *Root cause analysis: Simplified tools and techniques* (2nd ed.). Milwaukee, WI: ASQ Quality Press.
> Hodnett, E. (2010). Determine the root cause: 5 Whys. Six Sigma.

ASSIGNMENTS TO PRACTICE SKILL

Take on a tough and undoable project where others have failed. Besides analyzing the why behind the failure, think about what common characteristics are behind parallel situations that have succeeded.

If you're in a role with profit and loss responsibilities, switch to more of a staff role where you'll need to solve tough problems but with insufficient direct power to make anything happen. The politics of the job are usually sensitive and opposition is common.

Take responsibility for delivering a viable business strategy. The heavy strategic demands will necessitate finding the essence of the new direction you are proposing.

TAKE TIME TO REFLECT...

Here are some questions to reflect on as you focus on Essence. Think about how you might answer these today and how, through using the tips in this chapter, you might achieve a better result in the future.

When you're faced with a problem or challenge that's brand new, how much do you think about what the cause is before proposing or carrying out a solution?

Think about your last "aha" moment, when you had an insight or a realization about something. How would it feel if you could make those kinds of "ahas" and insights happen all the time?

How often do you have to return to the same problem again and again? When the first, second, and so on solutions failed? What is it about the problem that seems to make it unsolvable?

All truths are easy to understand once they are discovered; the point is to discover them.

Galileo Galilei
Italian philosopher, astronomer, and mathematician

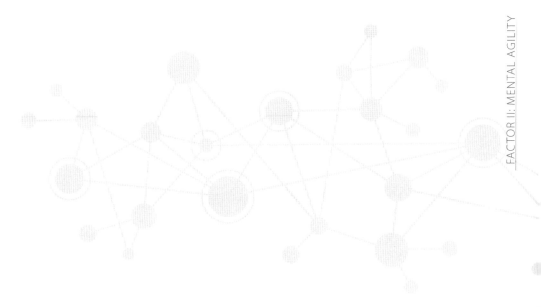

9

Complexity

In an era when globalization, disruptive technologies, world financial uncertainties, and population shifts/imbalances have become the norm, it's likely that the problems you face daily are becoming more and more complex. Success depends on figuring out the best solution to difficult, high-stakes issues. Issues that have so many moving parts that it's hard to make sense of it all. The person who can handle complexity isn't intimidated by it. Instead, he/she views complexity as a challenge, an intriguing puzzle—and one that he/she believes is solvable. Being skilled at Complexity means that when you're confronted with piles of information, often contradictory information, you are able to sort through, categorize, and distill the information down to simpler, understandable themes. Themes that you can draw upon to help solve not just the problem at hand but future, as yet unknown, problems.

I would not give a fig for the simplicity this side of complexity, but I would give my life for the simplicity on the other side of complexity.

Oliver Wendell Holmes
American Associate Justice of the Supreme Court of the United States

SKILLED

Can sift through complex data and information to make sense of it

Doesn't stop at obvious answers to problems

**Looks below surface qualities of situations
for underlying characteristics**

**Uses conceptual buckets to categorize complex situations
into simpler themes**

Can make sense of contradictory data

Describes the complex in simple, understandable ways

LESS SKILLED

Prefers to keep things uncomplicated

Has trouble conceptually sorting
disparate data into like themes

May be thrown by problems or
situations that are ambiguous

Easily frustrated when faced
with problems that have
many moving parts

May force comfortable solutions
to a problem that doesn't fit

Sticks to the obvious

OVERUSE OF SKILL

Exposes and explores every finite
detail before coming to a solution

Undervalues simple solutions

Makes things more complicated
than they need to be

Oversimplifies explanations

SOME POSSIBLE CAUSES OF LOWER SKILL

Causes help explain "why" a person may have trouble in this dimension. When seeking to increase skill, it's helpful to consider how these might play out in certain situations. And remember that all of these can be addressed if you are motivated to do so.

Doesn't think beyond own work/tasks

Gets frustrated when not "in the
know"

Gets stressed and overwhelmed easily

Not self-confident

Low tolerance for ambiguity and
uncertainty

Not comfortable with not knowing,
not answering; can't say "I don't know"

Overly results driven

DEVELOPMENTAL DIFFICULTY

When compared with other dimensions of Learning Agility, this dimension is **_moderately difficult_** to develop.

⭐ **Does It Best**

Galileo Galilei used visual thought experiments to explain his complex scientific theories. He described his relativity hypothesis this way: If two people are playing catch inside the cabin of a smooth-sailing ship, they can throw the ball back and forth with the same effort that it takes on land, regardless of the speed or direction of the ship.[10]

TIPS TO INCREASE SKILL IN COMPLEXITY

Prefer things that are uncomplicated?
Make the complex simple.

FOLLOW THE KEY STAGES OF COMPLEX PROBLEM SOLVING

Generally, problem solving starts with simplistic solutions to complex problems. First, everyone proposes a solution, even before there is a clear definition of the problem. The second stage is complexification. Someone always blows the issue out into its ultimate completeness with every finite detail exposed and explored. Many times it is correct, but usually also very involved. The third stage is parsimony—taking out all of the complexity and trimming down into the understandable. This last stage brings on simplicity which gets to the ultimate foundation of the issue, yielding an elegant and simple explanation or solution. It's important not to mistake simplistic for simple. The two may look alike, but simplistic solutions are usually incomplete and simple solutions are the accurate ones.

AVOID DRAWING PREMATURE CONCLUSIONS

Coming to quick, simple solutions is tempting but won't usually work for problems with either a lot of ambiguity or an overload of data. So resist the urge to just decide. Analyze the factors that cause you to avoid taking the time to consider complexity, and discipline yourself to spend half your problem-solving time defining the problem and thinking about all of its elements. Even if that's only ten minutes, use five to look more thoroughly. One way to do this: Ask how many elements or factors does this problem have? What is related to it? What is not related to it? If you're overwhelmed by complexity, put all like elements into conceptual buckets. For example, everything to do with costing in one bucket, everything having to do with people in another. Analyze how the buckets can work together and how they work against each other. Create processes for each bucket and processes for the buckets as a whole.

FACTOR II: MENTAL AGILITY

UNCOVER CAUSES OF COMPLEX PROBLEMS

Most issues worth considering are multicausal. Do you attribute cause and effect to relationships when you don't know if one causes the other? For example, if sales are down and we increase advertising and sales go up, this doesn't prove causality. They are simply related. Say we know that the relationship between sales and advertising is about the same as sales and number of employees. If sales go down, you probably wouldn't hire more people just based on that, so make sure one thing causes the other before acting on it. Ask why or how this could be a cause to better understand the nature of the beast. What would you accept as evidence that your problem definition is correct? What consequences would occur? What wouldn't occur? What are you prepared to do if your definition is incorrect?

Don't overcomplexify. Be sure to ask up front, Is there really more to this issue than meets the eye? Or is the solution self-evident? Don't force fit what is truly simple into a complex puzzle if it's not necessary.

RESOURCES TO LEARN MORE

Dettmer, H. W. (2007). *The logic thinking process: A systems approach to complex problem solving.* Milwaukee, WI: ASQ Quality Press.

Martin, R. (2007). *The opposable mind: How successful leaders win through integrative thinking.* Boston, MA: Harvard Business School Press.

10

Overwhelmed by complex problems? Pace yourself.

TAKE SMALL, INCREMENTAL STEPS

A key to not being overwhelmed by complexity is the tolerance of errors and mistakes, and absorbing the possible heat and criticism that follow. Acting on an ill-defined, complex problem with no precedents to follow means you need to experiment. People who are good at this are incrementalists. They make a series of smaller decisions, get instant feedback, correct the course, get a little more data, move forward a little more until the bigger problem is under control. They don't try to get it right the first time. Many problem-solving studies show that the second or third try is when we really understand the underlying dynamics of complex problems. Incrementalists also know that the more uncertain the situation is, the more likely it is they will make mistakes in the beginning. So start small so you can recover more quickly. And get used to the heat.

EXPAND SOLUTIONING OPTIONS THROUGH QUESTIONING

When faced with a complex challenge or problem, don't go to your past for the solution or conclusion first. Ask more questions up front. Not answers posing as questions with the only purpose being to confirm that your favorite past solution is the way to go. Probing, exploratory questions that reveal the complexity of the issue are needed to achieve the best solution. Studies have shown that about 50% of discussions involve answers; only 7% involve probing questions: Why does that work? Why might my solution not work this time? How would I know if it did or didn't? What's least likely? What's missing from the problem? Always ask the "what else could we do" question before settling on a solution.

 Don't completely discount your experience and abandon what's worked for you before. If you are facing a situation that has all the earmarks of situations where your favorite solutions have brought success in the past, simply pause to ask is this instance truly the same as before?

BALANCE TRYING FOR THE PERFECT ANSWER WITH ACTING ON A VIABLE OPTION

Many of us need or prefer to be 100% sure before acting. If you're worried about what people will say when you mess up, when every "t" isn't crossed, you're not alone. Perfectionism is tough to let go of because it's seen as a positive trait for most. When facing complexity, recognize your perfectionism for what it might be—collecting information to improve your confidence and avoid criticism, examining opportunities so long you miss them, or waiting for the perfect solution. Getting more information, raising question after question, won't ensure a fault-free decision and may actually be masking your aversion to risk. So be sure to find a balance between exposing and exploring problem complexity and landing on a workable solution.

RESOURCES TO LEARN MORE

Ackoff, R. L. (1978). *The art of problem solving: Accompanied by Ackoff's fables.* New York, NY: John Wiley & Sons, Inc.

McLeod, L. E. (2011, March 17). How to solve really big problems. *HuffingtonPost.com*

Ready to tackle complex problems?
Exercise your complexity muscle.

USE COMPLEX PROBLEM-SOLVING STRATEGIES

There are all kinds of mental exercises to increase your ability to manage complexity:

- Complex problems are hard to visualize. They tend to be either oversimplified or too complex to solve unless they are put in a visual format. Cut it up into its component pieces. Examine the pieces to see if a different order would help, or how you could combine three pieces into one.

- Another technique is a pictorial chart called a storyboard, where a problem is illustrated by its components being depicted as pictures.

- A variation of this is to tell stories that illustrate the +'s and –'s of a problem, then flowchart those according to what's working and not working. Another is a fishbone diagram used in Total Quality Management.

- Sometimes going to extremes helps. Adding every condition, every worst case you can think of sometimes will suggest a different solution. Taking the present state of affairs and projecting into the future may indicate how and where the system will break down.

GET UNSTUCK

If you're stumped trying to solve a complex problem, sleep on it. Take periodic breaks, whether stuck or not. This allows the brain to continue to work on the issue and releases the brain from reliance on past answers. Research shows that most breakthroughs come from our subconscious, when we're "not thinking about it." There's a reason Google and other highly innovative and creative companies actively encourage their employees to "play." These organizations understand that new insights don't usually come from a unifocus on the problem at hand. So put your problem away for a while. Once you've come up with every idea you can think of, throw them all out and wait for more to occur to you. Force yourself to forget about the issue and let your subconscious work on it for you.

USE DIVERSE RESOURCES

People-wise, find an expert or experts in your functional/technical/business area and go find out how they think and solve new, complex problems. Ask them what are the critical principles/drivers/things they look for. Have them tell you how they thought through a new problem in this area, the major skills they look for in sizing up people's proficiency in this area, key questions they ask about a problem, how they would suggest you go about learning quickly in this area. Reading-wise, fast-forward your thinking by reading publications like the *Futurist*, a journal of the World Future Society, or the *Popcorn Report* by Faith Popcorn. To better work through complexity requires having a broad perspective. In addition to knowing one thing well, it requires that you know at least a little about a lot of things.

RESOURCES TO LEARN MORE

de Bono, E. (1970). *Lateral thinking: Creativity step by step.* New York, NY: Harper & Row Publishers, Inc.

Friedman, S. (2008, April 11). A more holistic approach to problem solving. *Harvard Business Review.*

ASSIGNMENTS TO PRACTICE SKILL

Take on an assignment with heavy strategic demands, where you will be charting new ground, and collecting and analyzing lots of data.

Take on an assignment where the scope is substantially greater than what you do now, where you'll be juggling a high variety of activities. Your need to manage complexity and solve complicated, ambiguous problems will increase along with your workload.

Work on a team managing a significant business crisis (e.g., product scare, scandal, natural disasters, violent crime against employees, competitor significantly erodes market position) where you will need to make sense of a multitude of information in what could be a very time-sensitive setting.

TAKE TIME TO REFLECT...

Here are some questions to reflect on as you focus on Complexity. Think about how you might answer these today and how, through using the tips in this chapter, you might achieve a better result in the future.

What problems have you faced that were particularly complex? Where you felt overwhelmed by the sheer volume of information coming at you? What did you learn from these experiences that you would not have learned from a situation that was simplistic and easy?

In what areas would you consider yourself a perfectionist? Why do you value that? What would the impact be if you surrendered your need for certainty and embraced the uncertainty that comes with the complex?

Think back on the last month or so. When faced with new situations or problems, how often did your first thoughts turn to solutions or tactics you've used before? What's the risk of always applying the same tool, regardless of the fix needed?

Simplicity does not precede complexity, but follows it.

Alan Perlis
American computer scientist and recipient of the Turing Award

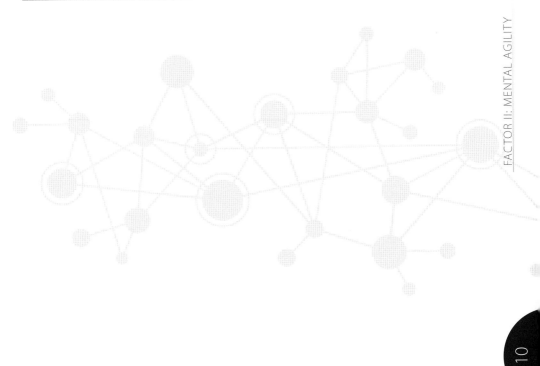

Manages
Uncertainty

11

It's likely that in your work and off-work life, you are constantly facing situations that are ambiguous or uncertain—where it's not clear what the problem is or what the solution is. Where the unknown outweighs the known by a wide margin. Some studies estimate that 90% of what managers deal with is at least somewhat ambiguous. The half-life of solutions, styles, or habits is getting shorter. Nothing lasts very long. In an era when clarity is scarce and certainty is fleeting, relying on solutions that have worked for you in the past is risky. Solving problems and getting things done in this volatile context means being willing to forge ahead when the path is foggy, at best. It means adjusting your approach—to both problems and people—to match changing conditions. To surrender the need to be sure. The world is getting less and less predictable. By having a mind-set geared to viewing uncertainty as the new normal, you will be better prepared when all those unknowns come your way.

The art of life is a constant readjustment to our surroundings.

Okakura Kakuzo
Japanese author and art critic

SKILLED
Comfortable when things are up in the air
Readily shifts approach or behavior to fit changing circumstances
Views uncertainty as the natural way of things
Can decide and act without having the total picture
Isn't paralyzed into inaction when the situation is ambiguous
Employs options and "what if" scenarios to navigate uncertainty

LESS SKILLED

May be uncomfortable
with ambiguity

Likes to stick to one action/solution,
rather than change course

Prefers to act when all the data are in

Operates best when things are
structured and predictable

Can't shift gears readily

Applies known, past solutions
to every problem

OVERUSE OF SKILL

May err toward the new and risky at
the expense of proven solutions

Doesn't honor others' need for some
level of clarity before acting

Undervalues orderly problem solving

Can be seen as too changeable;
appears inconsistent

SOME POSSIBLE CAUSES OF LOWER SKILL

Causes help explain "why" a person may have trouble in this dimension. When seeking to increase skill, it's helpful to consider how these might play out in certain situations. And remember that all of these can be addressed if you are motivated to do so.

Cautious

Dislikes change

Gets stressed or overwhelmed
easily

High need to close

Low frustration tolerance

Needs to be sure and certain

Prefers structure and control

Impatient

Can't multitask

DEVELOPMENTAL DIFFICULTY

When compared with other dimensions of Learning Agility, this dimension is **harder** to develop.

TIPS TO INCREASE SKILL IN MANAGES UNCERTAINTY

Holding on to certainty?
Give up control.

LET GO

Dealing comfortably with uncertainty and ambiguity means letting go of sureness. Like letting go of one trapeze in the air to catch the next one. For a small amount of time, you have hold of nothing but thin air. Taking that leap gets you to a new platform and a new place. If you hang on to the first trapeze, afraid you will fall, you will always return to the same old platform—safe but not new or different. And today and into the future, it's likely that your old, safe platform will keep getting smaller and smaller until it disappears completely. Manage the uncertainty around you by staying informed about business/technological change and ask what it means for your work. Visualize different outcomes. Talk about it. Invite ideas. The more you do this, the more comfortable you'll feel.

TRIM DOWN THE UNCERTAINTY

It turns out our brains are wired to dislike ambiguity even more than risk. Why? The brain craves certainty. Even when something is risky, risk is something identifiable, which makes it easier for our brains to process, evaluate, and assess the dangers. When things are highly ambiguous, the brain's defense center takes over. Any perceived loss of control kicks our threat system into high gear. The greater the sense of control, the quieter our brain's threat system becomes. So work to make the unknown known. Break it down into pieces. Identify it, set it aside, then work on the next unknown. Solve the little things and get them out of the way. Do something. Generally, little actions will trim the size of the uncertainty until it gets small enough to comfortably tackle.

STUDY PEOPLE WHO HAVE THRIVED UNDER CONDITIONS OF AMBIGUITY AND UNCERTAINTY

There are examples throughout history of people who have done well when the environment around them was highly ambiguous. People like Steve Jobs, Hillary Clinton, Winston Churchill, or Aung San Suu Kyi. Read their biographies or autobiographies. What did they do under time of high chaos? A helpful Web site for finding biographical summaries, books, videos, etc. is www.biography.com. Additionally, they list a monthly schedule for the Biography Channel, a cable channel on the A&E network dedicated to biography shows and specials on significant lives.

RESOURCES TO LEARN MORE

Robbins, M. (2010, September 13). 4 Simple ways to let go of control. *Huffington Post.*

Wilkinson, D. J. (2006). *The ambiguity advantage: What great leaders are great at.* Hampshire, England: Palgrave MacMillan.

Unsure how to navigate uncertainty?
Try different paths.

BALANCE THINKING WITH ACTION

Need or prefer or want to be 100% sure? Lots might prefer that. Perfectionism is tough to let go of because most people see it as a positive trait for themselves. Recognize your perfectionism for what it might be—collecting more information than others to improve your confidence in making a fault-free decision and, thereby, avoiding risk and criticism. Try to decrease your need for data and your need to be right all the time slightly every week until you reach a more reasonable balance between thinking it through and taking action. Try making some small decisions on little or no data. Anyone with 100% of the data can make good decisions. The real test is who can act the soonest with a reasonable amount, but not all, of the data.

DO QUICK EXPERIMENTS

When a situation has a lot of uncertainty to it and you're unsure how to proceed, be incremental. Instead of trying to tackle a highly ambiguous problem all at once, make some small decisions, get instant feedback, course correct as needed, and try again. That's what most successful innovators do. They try lots of quick, inexpensive experiments to increase their chances of success. They don't try to get it right the first time. They also know that the more uncertain the situation is, the more likely it is they will make mistakes in the beginning. Many problem-solving studies show that the second or third try is when we really understand the underlying dynamics of problems. Focus on those rather than your first.

11

BE PHILOSOPHICAL ABOUT FAILURE/CRITICISM

Most innovations fail, most proposals fail, most change efforts fail, anything worth doing takes repeated effort. To increase learning from your mistakes, design feedback loops to be as immediate as possible. The faster and the more frequent the cycles, the more opportunities to learn—if we do one smaller thing a day for three days instead of one bigger thing in three, we triple our learning opportunities. There will be many mistakes and failures; after all, since you're not sure, it's very likely no one else knows what to do either. They just have a right to comment on your errors. The best tack when confronted with a mistake is to say, "What can we learn from this?

 Learning from failures is key to effectively managing uncertainty, but it's just as important to know when it's time to quit or wait until there's enough information to have at least some chance of the solution being a winner. Be bold but don't be reckless.

RESOURCES TO LEARN MORE

Curiosity.com. (2011). Is it OK to fail? [Video file].

Gurvis, J., & Calarco, A. (2007). *Adaptability: Responding effectively to change.* Greensboro, NC: Center for Creative Leadership.

Freezing up under uncertainty?
Be more versatile.

DEVISE STRATEGIES TO DEAL WITH AMBIGUOUS SITUATIONS

All of us have to shift behavior each day. We act differently when things run well and when they don't. We act differently with different people. We act differently when things are settled and when conditions are uncertain. If you get sharp under pressure, use some humor to counter this tendency. If you're too tough on others, ask yourself how you'd like to be treated in this situation. Learn to recognize the clues that you're about to fall back on old behavior and be ready with a fresh strategy that you have decided in advance. If you know, for example, that a solution isn't working and you're likely to be questioned about it, be ready to engage others and get the benefit of their thinking.

DIAGNOSE YOUR TRANSITION TROUBLE SPOTS

To be able to adjust your approach effectively, you first need to understand which transitions trip you up. Study the transitions you make each day and write down which ones give you the most trouble and why. Are they more people related, process related, schedule related? Control your instant responses to shifts. Many of us respond to the fragmentation and discontinuities of work as if they were threats instead of the way life is. Sometimes our emotions and fears are triggered by switching from active to passive or soft to tough. This initial anxious response lasts 45–60 seconds, and we need to buy some time before we say or do something inappropriate. Research shows that, generally, the first thing we say or do isn't the best option. Practice holding back your first response long enough to think of other options. Manage your shifts, don't be a prisoner of them.

MANAGE UNCERTAINTY-DRIVEN STRESS

It's not uncommon to get stressed when dealing with increased ambiguity and uncertainty. We lose our anchor. We are not at our best when we are anxious, frustrated, upset, or when we lose our cool. Stress increases the chances that you will respond to conditions and people more emotionally. What brings out your emotional response? Write down why you get anxious: when you don't know what to do, don't want to make a mistake, afraid of the unknown consequences, don't have the confidence to act. When a highly ambiguous situation seems overwhelming, drop the problem for a while. Go do something else. Let your brain work on it while you do something safer.

> **RESOURCES TO LEARN MORE**
> Girard, K. (2009, May 4). Three tools to manage uncertainty. CBS News.
> Johri, V. (2010, March 9). Leaders today have to be comfortable with ambiguity. *Business Standard.*

ASSIGNMENTS TO PRACTICE SKILL

Increase the scope or complexity of what you are currently doing. This will automatically launch you out of your comfort zone and allow you to practice managing a high variety of activities where you won't know everything and will have to make decisions and solve problems when there isn't a clear path to follow.

Start something from scratch—something new and unique for you, your company, or customers. Some examples: building a new department, brand, or business unit; establishing a new location or new region; launching a new product or service. The very fact that this will be new for you will mean a lot of unknowns, ambiguity, and uncertainty for you to manage.

Work on a multifunctional team trying to solve an issue that crosses boundaries in the organization. Even better, make it an international assignment where you will be the outsider trying to navigate through a different culture, possible different language, and different expectations.

TAKE TIME TO REFLECT...

Here are some questions to reflect on as you focus on Manages Uncertainty. Think about how you might answer these today and how, through using the tips in this chapter, you might achieve a better result in the future.

Have you lost out on an opportunity for something great because you didn't feel comfortable acting on it without more sureness of the outcome? Was the sureness worth it? What would you have gained by taking a risk and deciding to do something, even when things were uncertain?

How comfortable are you in situations where you don't know the answers or the outcome? How do you respond to this? What could you do to be more effective?

Of the successes that you have achieved, which have been the most valuable to you? Why? Where did perseverance, fear, potential failure, mistakes, risk, and uncertainty come into play? How valuable would these successes have been to you if they were easily achieved? How does this shape your view on failure and mistakes?

11

The quest for certainty blocks the search for meaning. Uncertainty is the very condition to impel man to unfold his powers.

Erich Fromm
German psychoanalyst and social psychologist

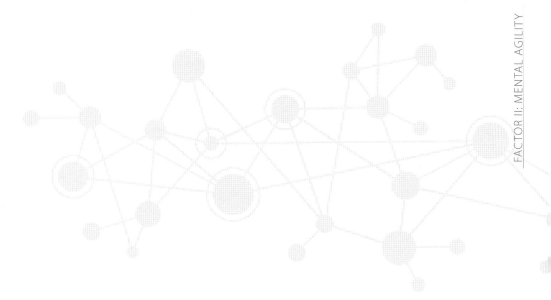

11

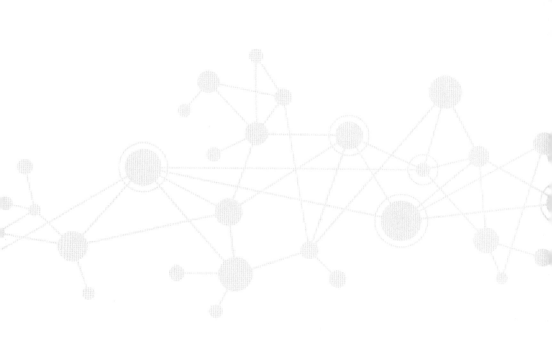

People Agility

People Agility is most certainly about being effective interpersonally, but it's much more than that. It's about taking a posture of openness, curiosity, and flexibility when it comes to relating to other people, seeking and collecting diverse opinions and viewpoints, and using the expanded understanding to achieve goals. People agile individuals show a genuine curiosity about other people and tend to be very observant and perceptive of others. The ability to anticipate how others are likely to act or respond helps people agile individuals adjust their own approach and how they communicate in different situations. With an eye toward achieving the best possible outcome for everyone involved, people agile individuals take a constructive approach to conflict by respectfully hearing out opposing positions, taking care not to incite or escalate conflict, and being open to having their minds and opinions altered by what they hear. One way people agile individuals measure their success is the degree to which they have a positive impact on others. This may be best reflected in how they take an interest and have a stake in other people's development and success. Not only do they share the spotlight, they bring out the best in others.

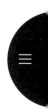

DIMENSIONS

Open Minded

People Smart

Situational Flexibility

Agile Communicator

Conflict Manager

Helps Others Succeed

Open Minded

Keeping an open mind is the willingness to postpone a decision or suspend judgment until you take in more information. It can also mean holding your own beliefs and opinions steady while agreeing to consider another point of view. Being Open Minded is not about being wishy-washy, relativistic, or not holding a solid set of beliefs. It's the ability to acknowledge that you are not right all the time, that you can learn from others, and that you will change your mind or your point of view when it makes sense to do so. Committed learners collect more viewpoints and are more open to ideas they don't necessarily agree with. The issue is what you can learn or gain from your experiences, not what you personally care to do or believe. Being open leads to more learning, being closed leads to less.

I would rather have a mind opened by wonder than closed by belief.

Gerry Spence
American lawyer and writer

12

SKILLED
Open to new and different ideas and solutions
Open to changing his/her mind
Recognizes, appreciates, and seeks to understand differences
Asks questions to learn more about other people
Is interested in what other people have to say
Tends to be more curious than judgmental about differences

LESS SKILLED
Only or most comfortable with those most like him/her

Dismisses different viewpoints

Prefers the company of like-minded people

Lacks curiosity and interest in different people's backgrounds and perspectives

Is unable or unwilling to look at things from another person's perspective

OVERUSE OF SKILL
May be perceived as a cultural tourist

Mistakes knowledge of differences for knowing others' experience

Loses sight of own identity and perspectives

SOME POSSIBLE CAUSES OF LOWER SKILL
Causes help explain "why" a person may have trouble in this dimension. When seeking to increase skill, it's helpful to consider how these might play out in certain situations. And remember that all of these can be addressed if you are motivated to do so.

Feels threatened by different beliefs or ideas

Wants to have it his/her own way

Narrow background and experiences

Not curious

Believes in one best solution

Inflexible or rigid

Too conventional

DEVELOPMENTAL DIFFICULTY
When compared with other dimensions of Learning Agility, this dimension is ***moderately difficult*** to develop.

⭐ Does It Best

In a country divided by deep-seated convictions, Abraham Lincoln emerged among several political opponents to be elected president of the United States in 1860. But rather than surrounding himself with like-minded men who would either concede to or align with his perspective on the country's issues, Lincoln appointed four of his most vehement critics to his cabinet. Many supporters questioned this decision but Lincoln replied, "We need the strongest men of the party in the Cabinet.... These were the strongest men. Then I had no right to deprive the country of their services." In her biography of Lincoln, Doris Kearns Goodwin chronicles how the president and these rivals with very different convictions worked together at a critical point in the history of the United States.[11]

TIPS TO INCREASE SKILL IN BEING OPEN MINDED

Is your worldview getting stale?
Find newness.

TAKE YOURSELF TO NEW PLACES

It's nice to have rituals and traditions, especially when it comes to your vacation plans. Maybe you have a family cabin, a favorite resort, or maybe you prefer the economical stay-cation. Consider shaking things up a bit and try somewhere new. Could be a road trip without a set itinerary that allows for stopping off at the occasional interesting shop or historical site. Could be exploring a part of the world you've never been to. Or why not explore a local neighborhood you've never visited? Chat with local residents, take in the sights, and pay attention to local media. Transport yourself out of your familiar surroundings and into less familiar places and perspectives. Ask yourself, What was I expecting? What surprised me? What does not appeal to me and why? What am I drawn to and why? How do I see things differently now?

STIMULATE YOUR SENSES

When was the last time you went to an art gallery, a concert, or a play? Experiencing the arts can wake up your mind, provide inspiration, and help you see things from a different angle. Art pushes the boundaries of our experience; it finds unconventional uses for objects or materials and new relationships between seemingly unrelated ideas. Notice what pieces resonate with you and which ones don't. Ask yourself why. Look at the pieces from the artist's perspective. What was the artist trying to accomplish? How does it fit with other works? Explore your emotional response to what you experienced. What triggered the way you felt? And how do the arts expand your thinking?

12

DO SOMETHING THAT SCARES YOU A LITTLE BIT

Opening ourselves up to new experiences and new ideas often involves overcoming some fear. It's useful that humans have evolved to be scared of certain things that could hurt us. But irrational fears we've added along the way may be based on incomplete or inaccurate information. To confront these fears, it helps to check assumptions. Are you scared to raise your hand for a tough assignment because you might fail? Do you feel hesitant to introduce yourself to someone because you might get the brush-off? What risks can you take to prove to yourself that your fears may be overblown?

RESOURCES TO LEARN MORE

Cutts, M. (2011, July). Try something new for 30 days [Video file].

Lickerman, A. (2010, April 1). Trying new things. *Psychology Today.*

Think you have all the answers?
Get a dose of humility.

ADMIT IT WHEN YOU DON'T KNOW

A simple way to practice opening your mind to new information and ideas is to start with the statement, "I don't know." Then try following that with a question: What do you think? Who should I ask? How could I learn more? We are trained to sound authoritative and confident at work. In many cases, assuredness is what is rewarded. But you know the difference between speaking from experience and making something up. There is nothing wrong with venturing a guess—just do yourself a favor and admit that's what you're doing. Once you say, "I don't know for sure," you open your mind up to learning more.

FIND A BIGGER EXPERT

No matter how knowledgeable you are about a topic, unless you are the world's leading authority on that topic, there is someone else you can learn from. Find the most prominent thought leaders in your field, read their columns or studies, reflect on how their wisdom and experience expands your own understanding. Better yet, find some respected authorities whose opinions and conclusions diverge from your own. What are they seeing that you're not? How would you explain the evidence that is contrary to your own theories? What part of their rationale would you adopt? How does this new information alter your thinking?

GET A SPARRING PARTNER

Whether it's a teacher, a mentor, a colleague, or a spouse, finding someone who can help you scrutinize your thinking and your approach can help open your mind. Trusted thought partners can focus on the problem, play devil's

12

advocate, and keep things from getting personal or adversarial. Take the time to wrestle with ideas, poke holes in different solutions, and uncover faulty assumptions. Ask them: What am I not considering? Where is my reasoning off? Are there possible unintended consequences that I am not seeing? What would be a better route to take?

RESOURCES TO LEARN MORE

LinkedIn Discussion Forums. (2011, August 25.) How to stay objective when facing conflict between team members? Linkedin.com

Peale, N. V. (2011). *The power of positive thinking.* Bronx, NY: Ishi Press International. (Original work published 1952.)

Finding yourself in unknown territory?
Suspend judgment.

ALLOW YOURSELF TO BE SURPRISED

It's normal to have a set of expectations, a clear idea of how you want things to play out, a preconceived notion of who you can rely on for help. The question is, how receptive are you to the occasional surprise? Do you stay open and see what's new? Do you quickly try to go back to the plan? By allowing yourself to be surprised, you may find that you reach an even better destination. You can even take it a step further and seek out surprises. Ask for opinions from people you do not normally consult—you might learn something new. Bring in more team members to collaborate on a tough challenge—the best solution may arise spontaneously from dialogue. Surprises may seem risky, but the payoff for giving up a little control can be very rewarding.

LISTEN AND THINK BEFORE YOU DISMISS

During conversations, it's easy to spend your time evaluating and discounting other people's viewpoints. Often, people focus their energy on preparing how they will refute or dispute what the other person is saying. Rather than convincing everyone else that you are right, take a moment to stay neutral and understand those other viewpoints. How did they form their opinions? What leads them to a conclusion that is different from yours? If you were in their shoes, would you have come to the same conclusion as they did? By pausing the debate and seeking to understand, you not only build empathy for the other person's perspective, you know more precisely how and why you differ on the topic.

Don't let neutrality tip into indifference. While it is virtuous to be a neutral, objective party, most of our work requires us to land on a point of view, a way forward, a recommended approach. If you hang out in neutral too long and view everything as relative, you might lose your opportunity to get something done.

THINK IN POSSIBILITY

Before you dismiss something as impossible, think about what is possible. Before you say no, think about what you can say yes to. Redirecting our minds to think in possibility open us up to options we had not considered. Think about how many times throughout history that explorers and scientists, athletes and political leaders have been told, "That's impossible." What if everyone listened to these external or internal voices drawing limits on what can be. What impossible accomplishments will you witness in your lifetime? What have you accomplished that you wouldn't have thought possible?

RESOURCES TO LEARN MORE

Johnson, K. (2012, May 31). Get to know people [Video file].

Lawler, E. E., III. (2003). *Treat people right: How organizations and individuals can propel each other into a virtuous spiral of success.* San Francisco, CA: Jossey-Bass.

ASSIGNMENTS TO PRACTICE SKILL

Volunteer to work for a charity or community organization to build your experiences with a broader spectrum of people—for example, younger or older than you, different cultures, different neighborhoods, or different economic status.

Lead a project or task force where the other people in the group are towering experts but you aren't. You will need to gain an understanding of their viewpoints on the subject and leverage those to be successful.

Manage a dissatisfied internal or external customer where moving from conflict to satisfaction or collaboration is crucial. Play out the situation from the customer's viewpoint—you're likely to unearth common ground and a better understanding of what is behind their dissatisfaction.

12

TAKE TIME TO REFLECT...

Here are some questions to reflect on as you focus on being Open Minded. Think about how you might answer these today and how, through using the tips in this chapter, you might achieve a better result in the future.

What would it look like if you focused less on convincing others of your opinion or perspective and more on listening to theirs?

Where might your expertise prevent you from learning and growing?

How do you ensure that you have not become so set in your ways or ideas that you are not open to new experiences and learning from them?

....

Travel is fatal to prejudice, bigotry, and narrow-mindedness.

Mark Twain
American humorist, satirist, lecturer, and writer

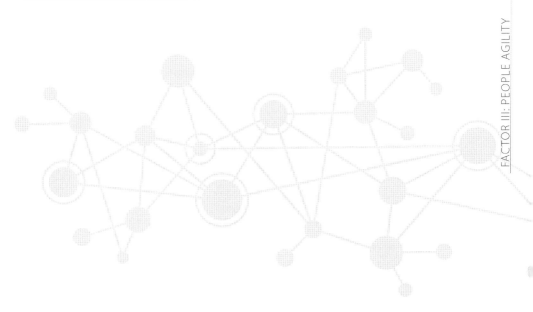

12

People
Smart

Being People Smart allows you to be one step ahead because you can accurately anticipate how people are likely to respond in different situations. It's a combination of sizing up people's qualities and discerning what makes them that way. What it's *not* is about relying on a set of stereotypes or shortcuts. If you are People Smart, you read individuals almost intuitively. You zero in on what makes the other person unique. You are quickly in tune with their strengths and weaknesses, their values, their perspectives. Your skilled observation, empathy, and gained insight put you in a privileged position. You clearly understand who you are interacting with, what they care most about, and how they are likely to think, feel, and act. This ability to forecast comes in handy in all kinds of interpersonal situations. You have the people knowledge necessary to help you adjust and respond appropriately. You are better equipped to develop others' weaknesses or leverage their strengths. You can make better hiring decisions. The list of benefits goes on and on.

You are one of the rare people who can separate
your observation from your perception...
you see what is, where most people see what they expect.

Tsitsi Dangarembga
Zimbabwean author and filmmaker

FACTOR III: PEOPLE AGILITY

SKILLED

Understands what makes people the way they are

Is able to forecast how people will act

Sizes up an audience quickly

Reads people well

Can articulate the qualities, perspectives, strengths, and weaknesses of others

LESS SKILLED

Doesn't know why people act the way they do

Misreads others

Is caught off guard by others' actions and reactions

Slow to pick up on social cues or body language

OVERUSE OF SKILL

Is preoccupied with trying to anticipate everyone else's behavior

Reads too much into others' behavior

Makes others feel self-conscious

Insights about other people are static; is not open to new or changing evidence

SOME POSSIBLE CAUSES OF LOWER SKILL

Causes help explain "why" a person may have trouble in this dimension. When seeking to increase skill, it's helpful to consider how these might play out in certain situations. And remember that all of these can be addressed if you are motivated to do so.

Doesn't care about others

Narrow people background

Prefers to be alone

Not observant

Sees people in too simple terms

Self-centered

Too quick to judge

Uses stereotypes

Doesn't listen

13

DEVELOPMENTAL DIFFICULTY

When compared with other dimensions of Learning Agility, this dimension is **harder** to develop.

Did You Know?

Halos, Warts, and All: When someone leaves a strong impression on us (whether positive or negative), it's common to generalize that impression to all aspects of the person's personality, behaviors, and skills. Psychologists call this the "Halo Effect."[12] While it's possible that someone who is arrogant is also dishonest or that someone who presents well is organized, it is an unfair assumption to make the leap without evidence. Having clear criteria and paying close attention to actual behavior lessens the chance of perceiving something that isn't necessarily there. Someone who is People Smart avoids extrapolating and sees people as they are—halos, warts, and all.

TIPS TO INCREASE SKILL IN BEING PEOPLE SMART

Having trouble seeing it from their perspective?
Build your ability to empathize.

SEE PEOPLE, THE ROLE THEY PLAY, AND THE VALUE THEY BRING

This may seem elementary, but the first step toward being more People Smart is to see people. In the rush of daily life, we are often focused on "I": on what *I* need, where *I* am going, and whether *I* am going to be late. Our focus on ourselves can prevent us from noticing or considering other people. Practice seeing people. What role do they play? How are their needs being met or not met? What value do they bring to the world? By taking a moment to consider other people's place in the world and their experience, you can build empathy—the ability to understand and be aware of the feelings, thoughts, and experiences of others.

TREAT PEOPLE AS INDIVIDUALS, NOT MEMBERS OF A GROUP

Most people do not like being lumped into a group unless there are allowances made for exceptions to the rule. Variation within a group is bigger than variation between groups. People's identities are complex and sometimes paradoxical. Viewing someone merely as part of a larger demographic strips away meaningful layers of their identity and leaves you with a very superficial (and possibly inaccurate) understanding of who they are and what they care about. Think about the incomplete picture other people would get of you if they only had a few key data points about you—gender, race, profession, place of residence. Of course, these are important aspects of identity, but there is so much more that makes each of us unique individuals. Find out what makes other people unique.

TAKE TIME TO GET TO KNOW PEOPLE

There is a simple way to learn about what drives people, what their career aspirations are, what their strengths and weaknesses are. Get to know them. Take a moment to elevate the conversation from everyday tactics and get a broader picture of who you work next to every day. Don't assume you already know. And be ready to share the same information about yourself. Building more personal relationships takes time. You may not feel that you have much time to spare, but understanding who you work with can help you figure out whom to call upon when you need support or assistance later on.

RESOURCES TO LEARN MORE
Johnson, K. (2012, May 31). Get to know people [Video file].

Lawler, E. E., III. (2003). *Treat people right: How organizations and individuals can propel each other into a virtuous spiral of success.* San Francisco, CA: Jossey-Bass.

Want to read people more accurately?
Become a master observer.

BECOME A STUDENT OF THE PEOPLE AROUND YOU

Beyond basic intelligence and personality, what qualities do you notice in the people around you? What do you think their key strengths are and why? How do you see others working around their weaknesses? By taking the time to outline some key strengths and weaknesses, you are naming the skills and making those skills easier to observe in action. Look deeper than typical descriptors like smart, capable, talented, personable. What specifically does a person do that warrants those descriptions? The better you are at sizing up and describing other people's skills, the better you will be able to match the right person to a business need.

LISTEN TO WHAT IS BEING SAID AND WHAT IS NOT BEING SAID

So much is communicated without words. Hence the phrase "read between the lines." Next time you're watching your favorite show or movie, hit the mute button and see what you're able to decipher. What emotions are at play? What underlying motivations are driving each person? What's the mood of the room? What interpersonal dynamics are you picking up on? When you turn the volume back up, what are you hearing? Notice if there is a discrepancy between the verbal and non-verbal cues. You are now practicing the art of careful observation.

 It's true that non-verbals carry a lot of meaning, but be careful not to add too much meaning to a gesture or a look. And don't always assume the worst or take things personally. What you see as a disrespectful eye roll may be someone adjusting a contact lens.

13

PRACTICE EVALUATING OTHERS

Whether you raise your hand to be part of an interview panel or you take extra time to complete a multi-rater assessment, evaluating people will develop your ability to read other people more accurately and objectively. Structured interviews and assessments provide you with clear criteria to compare the person against. And in the process of assessing one person, you can be comparing that person to other people you work with. If there are questions you have trouble answering because you haven't observed that skill or behavior, make a note to pay closer attention next time you see the person in action. Evaluating others can help you articulate and fine-tune your perceptions of others.

RESOURCES TO LEARN MORE

Dimitrius, J., & Mazzarella, W. P. (2008). *Reading people: How to understand people and predict their behavior: Anytime, anyplace.* New York, NY: Ballantine Books.

Must Read Summaries. (2011). *Summary: How to win friends and influence people — Dale Carnegie* [Kindle edition].

Are you off in your people predictions? Take time to investigate.

CHECK YOUR ASSUMPTIONS BY ASKING QUESTIONS

If on a regular basis you find yourself surprised by how people act or react, consider gathering more information before you make a guess. Whether you have bad news to share or something sensitive to discuss, talk to a trusted colleague about the future interaction. Ask the colleague how they think the other person will respond, where the other person's mind-set might be, and how the person might be feeling. Ask what you can do to be considerate of where the person is coming from, how you might approach the conversation differently. During the interaction, take time to ask the other person questions that will help you clarify how they are doing, why they see something a certain way. Of course, implied in this suggestion is that after asking the questions, you listen.

GET OUT OF YOUR PEOPLE COMFORT ZONE

If you find that you are consistently drawn to people who are like you, branch out and seek some variety in the people you associate with. When you spend most of your time with people who have similar skills, political views, background, and personality, you are limiting how much you can understand about other people. Strike up conversations with people you don't know or wouldn't normally talk to or maybe even people who annoy you for some reason. Turn off your judgment for a moment and work on understanding them better. You are likely to learn from your differences.

REVIEW AND DISSECT
Were you sure an interaction would go one way and it went another? Did you make a bet on a new hire that did not pan out? Understanding the discrepancy between your expectations and reality can keep you from getting caught off guard in the future. Process and dissect what happened. Why were you surprised? What clues did you ignore? What questions did you forget to ask? Did you ignore disconfirming evidence and only pay attention to things that confirmed your preconceived ideas? Learning from these misjudgments or bad calls can help you hone your people prediction skills and flag potential judgment errors next time.

> **RESOURCES TO LEARN MORE**
> Dimitrius, J., & Mazzarella, W. P. (2008). *Reading people: How to understand people and predict their behavior: Anytime, anyplace.* New York, NY: Ballantine Books.
> Segal, J., & Jaffe, J. (2008). *The language of emotional intelligence: The five essential tools for building powerful and effective relationships.* New York, NY: McGraw Hill.

ASSIGNMENTS TO PRACTICE SKILL
Resolve a conflict between two people or two departments. Get clear on the values and positions of each individual and gauge how that will play out during resolution efforts.

Volunteer to help recruiting at the annual job fair. Through informal conversation, begin to pick up on what individuals' strengths and weaknesses are.

Assemble a team of diverse people to accomplish a difficult task. Plan how to leverage individuals based on the unique value each person brings to the team.

13

TAKE TIME TO REFLECT...

Here are some questions to reflect on as you focus on being People Smart. Think about how you might answer these today and how, through using the tips in this chapter, you might achieve a better result in the future.

> When have you been too quick to form a judgment about someone that was later unfounded? What did you learn from that experience?

Where is your team particularly talented? How can you find out about talents your team members may have that you don't already know about? How can you leverage this existing talent?

> When have you been caught by surprise at the amount of resistance to a change or an idea? What did you learn about the people involved?

I must try to see the difference between my picture of a person and his behavior, as it is narcissistically distorted, and the person's reality as it exists regardless of my interests, needs and fears.

Erich Fromm
German psychoanalyst and social psychologist

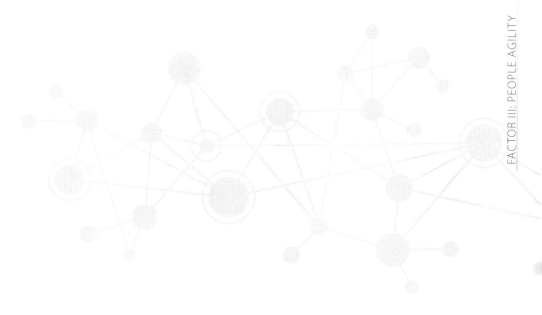

13

Situational
Flexibility

Those who are highly people agile are well versed in the interpersonal give-and-take required for different situations. They recognize that there is always a need to adapt and show up differently because no two situations are exactly alike. You wouldn't behave the same way in a politically charged board meeting as you would in a leadership team brainstorming session. Being skilled in Situational Flexibility means you are in tune with subtle differences between various interpersonal situations and you can adjust and fine-tune your behavior to what fits best. This does not mean that you are being disingenuous or inauthentic. You simply understand the advantage of bringing certain qualities to the foreground. You bring more empathy in times of stress and change, more direction in times of uncertainty, more diplomacy in times of conflict. And you continuously gauge the impact you are having, ready to make further adjustments to your demeanor and approach. You do not automatically choose your default preferences; instead, you pay attention to what each situation requires of you and adjust accordingly.

You must be shapeless, formless, like water.
When you pour water in a cup, it becomes the cup.
When you pour water in a bottle, it becomes the bottle.
When you pour water in a teapot, it becomes the teapot.
Water can drip and it can crash. Become like water my friend.

Bruce Lee
Chinese American actor, martial arts cultural icon, and film director and producer

SKILLED

Reads the room and responds to the demands of the situation

Can sense interpersonal dynamics

Adjusts to situations in real time

Sees situations from different points of view

Can play different roles depending on the circumstances

Picks up on subtle cues and adjusts

LESS SKILLED

Acts the same, regardless of the situation

Doesn't pick up on or ignores situational cues

Less in tune with interpersonal or political dynamics

Expects others to adjust to his/ her preferred style and approach

OVERUSE OF SKILL

Is overly accommodating to the needs of the situation

Comes across as waffling

May appear inauthentic or manipulative; panders

May be overly concerned with others' perceptions

SOME POSSIBLE CAUSES OF LOWER SKILL

Causes help explain "why" a person may have trouble in this dimension. When seeking to increase skill, it's helpful to consider how these might play out in certain situations. And remember that all of these can be addressed if you are motivated to do so.

Has a preferred style

Ignores politics

Oblivious to sensitive dynamics

Prefers simple, straightforward situations

Focused on own agenda

Doesn't want to concede anything

Subscribes to "I am what I am"

Out of touch

Thinks he/she is above it all

Acts primarily out of self-interest

Unable to see the bigger picture

14

DEVELOPMENTAL DIFFICULTY

When compared with other dimensions of Learning Agility, this dimension is **harder** to develop.

135

⭐ Does It Best

Rock star, business partner, philanthropist, and political activist. U2's Bono wears many hats. Whether he's on tour or at a charity event, he is arresting and dynamic. As a business partner, he is shrewd. As a philanthropist, he is empathetic and creative—seeking ways to raise money to fight poverty and disease. As for his political activism, Bono is respectful and focused on dialogue when he meets with world leaders to discuss debt relief and other humanitarian efforts. And, while he didn't begin his career with the ability to play all of these roles, he has gradually grown comfortable in situations as varied as guest editing an issue of *Vanity Fair,* launching (PRODUCT)$^{RED™}$ with iconic global brands, collaborating with a diverse list of artists and writers, and graciously receiving countless awards for his music as well as his humanitarian work.[13]

TIPS TO INCREASE SKILL IN SITUATIONAL FLEXIBILITY

No filter?
Stop and think.

THINK ABOUT THE CONSEQUENCES

Use mental rehearsal to think about different ways you could engage and then picture the response. Try to see yourself acting in opposing ways to get the same thing done—when to be tough, when to let others decide, when to deflect the issue because it's not ready to be decided. What cues would you look for to select an approach that matches what you want to accomplish? Imagine trying to get the same thing done with two different groups with two different approaches. How do they play out in your mind? Now focus on the situation at hand and the players involved—which approach will likely yield the best outcome?

PRACTICE SELF-CONTROL

If you have trouble controlling your instant reactions, press the pause button. Many of us respond to situations as if they were threats instead of the way life is. Sometimes our emotions and fears are triggered when we switch from active to passive or soft to tough. This initial anxious response lasts 45–60 seconds, and we need to buy some time before we say or do something inappropriate. Research shows that, generally, somewhere between the second and third thing you think to say or do is the best option. Practice holding back your first response long enough to think of a second and a third. Rather than react, adapt and thoughtfully respond to situations instead.

14

TAKE A PAUSE

Before you jump in with your typical approach to a situation, stall for a moment to see what you're missing. Gather more information, listen, try to get a read on others in the room. People who can adjust to any situation have a bag of techniques they use. They give reasons for everything they say, saving any solution statements for last. They ask lots of questions, speak briefly, summarize often, and, when disagreeing, they put it in conditional terms ("I don't think so, but what do you think?"). The point of these is to elicit as much information about the reactions of others as they can. They are loading their files so they can change behavior when needed.

RESOURCES TO LEARN MORE

DiSalvo, D. (2011). *What makes your brain happy and why you should do the opposite.* Amherst, NY: Prometheus Books.

Guilmartin, N. (2009). *The power of pause: How to be more effective in a demanding, 24/7 world.* San Francisco, CA: Jossey-Bass.

Trouble shifting gears?
Practice the transitions.

LEARN TO TRANSITION COMFORTABLY BETWEEN SITUATIONS

As one song says, "I want to be me." Not many of us have that luxury. Each situation we deal with is a little bit, somewhat, or a lot different. In order to be truly effective across situations and people, we are called upon to act differently. In control at 9 a.m., following at 10 a.m., quiet at 11 a.m., and dominating at noon. It's all in a day's work. Respectful with the boss, critiquing with peers, caring for directs, and responding to customers. No trickery. No blowing with the wind. No Machiavellianism. Just adjusting flexibly to the demands of each situation. Work on first reading the situation and the people. Monitor your gear-shifting behavior for a week at work and at home. What switches give you the most trouble? The least? Why? Off-work, practice gear-shifting transitions. Go from a civic meeting to a water fight with your kids, for example. On the way between activities, if only for a few seconds, think about the transition you're making and the frame of mind needed to make it work well.

If you find yourself making wild swings in personality between different interactions and situations, stop to ask yourself if you are focusing too much on accommodating others and not enough on being yourself. If you adjust too much, people may perceive that you are inconsistent and waffling, or even worse—inauthentic and manipulative.

14

TACKLE WHAT'S TOUGHEST FOR YOU

Which transitions are the toughest for you? Write down the five toughest for you. What do you have a hard time switching to and from? Use this knowledge to assist you in making a list of discontinuities (tough transitions) you face, such as:

· Confronting people vs. being approachable and accepting

· Leading vs. following

· Going from firing someone to a business-as-usual staff meeting

Write down how each of these discontinuities makes you feel and what you may do that gets you in trouble. For example, you may not shift gears well after a confrontation or you may have trouble taking charge again after passively sitting in a meeting all day. Create a plan to attack each of the tough transitions.

GAUGE YOUR IMPACT AND ADJUST

One way to gauge your impact is to ask people for direct feedback on what you are doing while you are doing it and immediately after. People are often reluctant to give you feedback, especially negative or corrective information. Generally, to get it, you must ask for it. If people are reluctant to give criticism, help by making self-appraisal statements rather than asking questions. Saying, "I think I talked too long on that topic in the meeting, what do you think?" is easier for most people to reply to than a question which asks them to volunteer this point. Once you get the feedback, do something with it. Adjust and adapt to be more effective in that situation.

RESOURCES TO LEARN MORE

Burton, K. (2010). *Live life, love work.* West Sussex, England: Capstone Publishing Ltd.

Gurvis, J., & Calarco, A. (2007). *Adaptability: Responding effectively to change.* Greensboro, NC: Center for Creative Leadership.

Comfortable with who you are?
Stretch yourself.

PULL BACK ON OVERUSED SKILLS

If it's your default mode, it's probably something you overapply. A lot of us overdo some of our strengths. We push for results too hard. We analyze data too long. We try to be too nice. For those overdone behaviors, it's difficult for us to do the opposite. Find out what you overdo by getting feedback, either a 360° feedback instrument or by polling your closest associates. Find out how adaptable people think you are when under pressure and how well you handle the fragmentation of a typical day. Try to balance your behavior against whatever you overdo. Don't replace what you do—add to it. If you

14

get brusque under pressure, take three deep breaths and consciously slow down or use some humor. If you're too tough, ask yourself how you'd like to be treated in this situation. If you run over others, tell them what you're thinking about doing and ask them what they think should be done. Strengths become overused skills when you use them, regardless of the situation. Be more precise and adjust to the specific need.

GO FOR MORE VARIETY
Get out of your comfort zone. Put yourself in very different situations than you typically encounter. Raise your hand for volunteer assignments that represent a new challenge. Set tasks for yourself that force you to shift gears, such as being a spokesperson for your organization when tough questions are expected, making peace with an enemy, or managing people who are novices at a task. If you already have these tasks as part of your job, use them to observe yourself and try new behaviors. Experiencing a variety of situations will help you become more flexible and adaptable.

LAUGH AT YOURSELF
Whether you do this in private or in public, having a sense of humor about yourself only serves to humanize you. Funny stories about situations where you were embarrassed, did the exact wrong thing, fumbled a well-rehearsed line, or committed a faux pas are opportunities to learn while entertaining yourself and others. Perfection is never the goal, only learning and improving along the way.

> **RESOURCES TO LEARN MORE**
> AttitudeTVChannel. (2010, May 9). Sam Glenn's airplane story [Video file].
> Kaplan, R. E., & Kaiser, R. B. (2009, February). Stop overdoing your strengths. *Harvard Business Review, 87*(2), 100–103.

14

ASSIGNMENTS TO PRACTICE SKILL
Take on a tough and undoable project where there are no clear answers or paths to completion. Figuring things out as you go will probably require resourcefulness and a willingness to wear multiple hats in a variety of situations.

Go on a business trip to a foreign country you've not been to before. Meeting your hosts for the first time and acclimating yourself to the various social and business events will require Situational Flexibility.

Help people infuse humor into their presentations. Adept use of humor requires a good understanding of the audience, what will play, what would go over their heads, what would fall flat. Think through the situation and find the best way to incorporate a light touch.

TAKE TIME TO REFLECT...

Here are some questions to reflect on as you focus on Situational Flexibility. Think about how you might answer these today and how, through using the tips in this chapter, you might achieve a better result in the future.

Think about a time when you were placed in a situation where you did not already know what to do or how to get things done. How did you go about learning in real time? What did you do to manage the situation effectively? What did you learn about yourself?

Think about a situation where you resisted adjusting your approach when you would have been better served by adapting to it. What was it that prevented you from adapting earlier? How will this same obstacle be present in the future? What will you do differently?

When was it beneficial for you to adjust to a situation. What helped your decision making and subsequent action in that situation? How can you apply that learning to other situations for future success?

14

....

It is a wise person that adapts themselves to all contingencies; it's the fool who always struggles like a swimmer against the current.

Anonymous

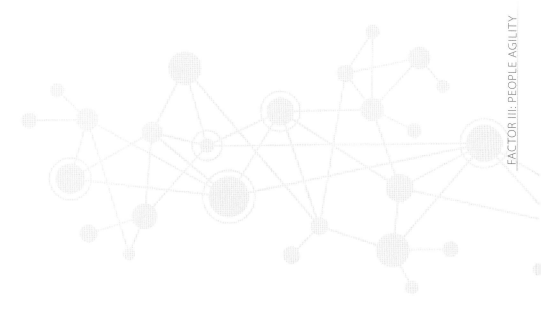

Agile
Communicator

The act of communicating, by definition, involves more than one person. Agile communicating is as much about the content, the *what*, of the message as it is about the *how* of the process. Acquiring information, or the what, of a topic is usually pretty straightforward and usually only involves you. The how is where Learning Agility shows up. Communicating what you know or communicating so you can get done what you need to get done means reading and responding to others, both in advance and in the moment. This means adjusting your pace, style, and message to the audience, whether you're communicating one-on-one or one-to-many. When you communicate what you know in a way others will understand, it's more likely that your message will not only get through but will achieve the impact you're looking for. Knowing it yourself is seldom enough. Knowing how to convey meaning to others so that *they* know it equals success.

Everyone hears only what he understands.

Johann Wolfgang von Goethe
German playwright, poet, novelist, and dramatist

15

SKILLED

Considers the audience

Is articulate

Communicates the complex so others can understand

Uses appropriate language to sell a view

Fairly presents the arguments of others

LESS SKILLED	OVERUSE OF SKILL
Doesn't adjust to audience needs or preferences	May be so responsive to audience that key message is lost
Unable to simplify a complex argument	May appear to not hold a strong point of view
Always presents the same way	Comes across as condescending by oversimplifying the message
May not accurately restate the case of others	
May overwhelm audience with emotion or detail	

SOME POSSIBLE CAUSES OF LOWER SKILL

Causes help explain "why" a person may have trouble in this dimension. When seeking to increase skill, it's helpful to consider how these might play out in certain situations. And remember that all of these can be addressed if you are motivated to do so.

Has trouble empathizing	Inflexible or rigid
Doesn't listen	Unable to react quickly
Impatient	Has difficulty reading others' verbal and nonverbal cues
Lacks focus	

15

DEVELOPMENTAL DIFFICULTY

When compared with other dimensions of Learning Agility, this dimension is **_moderately difficult_** to develop.

⭐ **Does It Best**

Former U.S. president Bill Clinton connects with his audience by personally relating to them. When addressing a citizen's question about the economy in a 1992 presidential election debate, Clinton replied, "Being governor of a small state, when people lose their jobs, there's a good chance I'll know them by name; when a factory closes, I'll know the person who ran it; when the businesses go bankrupt, I know them."[14] In that one statement, Clinton seamlessly demonstrated understanding while reinforcing his role as a leader. (Arkansas state governor at the time.)

TIPS TO INCREASE SKILL AS AN AGILE COMMUNICATOR

Think there's only one way to communicate with others? Read your audiences.

COMMUNICATE OUTSIDE IN, NOT INSIDE OUT
Select your communication approach from the other person in, not from you out. Your best choice of approach should be determined by the other person or group, not you. When crafting and delivering messages, don't default to what you want to do or what would make you happy or is easiest for you. Instead, ask yourself, What are the demand characteristics of this situation? How does this person or audience best learn? Which of my approaches or styles would work best? How can I best accomplish my goals? How can I alter my approach and tactics to be the most effective? Think about communicating as if the other person or the group were customers you wanted. How would you craft an approach?

CATCH A CUE
Verbal cues are easy to spot. They often come in the form of questions, either reinforcing of your message or challenging to oppose it. Non-verbals are tougher but can be even more revealing. The general research on communication indicates that more than 50% of communication power comes from visual cues. Head nods, eye contact, affirming sounds, energetic leaning forward, or even a relaxed stance usually mean your message is getting through the way you intended. On the flip side, frowning, head shaking, and body agitation can be signs of either opposition to the message or a need for more clarity. Fascination with the contents of one's mobile device probably means either the content or delivery of your message isn't compelling enough to overcome multi-taskism. Study up on the cues people give you that let you know your message is getting across (or not).

15

CRAFT AN ADAPTABLE MESSAGE

Any single communication approach will generally not play equally well across different audiences. Many times, you will have to adjust the tone, pace, style, and even the message and how you couch it for different audiences. If you are communicating the same message to multiple audiences, always ask yourself how are they different? Some common questions to consider are: What's their time tolerance? How much do they expect to participate? Do they prefer formal or informal? Would they rather just chat about the topic? How sophisticated is the group? How much pushback do you expect? Will a logical or emotional argument play better? Determine the answers to these questions and adjust accordingly.

RESOURCES TO LEARN MORE

Brown, P. B. (2006, September 2). Listen up. Know your audience. *New York Times*.

Navarro, J. (2008). *What every body is saying: An ex-FBI agent's guide to speed-reading people*. New York, NY: Harper-Collins.

Think knowing it is the same as communicating it?
Connect to communicate.

KEEP IT (JUST) SIMPLE ENOUGH

When you know a lot about something, it's tempting to describe it to others at the level of your own understanding. Though you may be the expert, communicating is not about showing how smart you are. It's about getting your message across so that others can understand as well. Don't try to tell the audience all you know, even if they are well informed on the topic. Drowning people in detail can lose even the most knowledgeable and interested. To appeal to your entire audience, use straightforward language and logic. Watch out for jargon if you have to explain something complex. If you are speaking on a technical issue to a non-technical audience, use metaphors or examples from everyday life that you're sure the audience can identify with.

 Be careful not to oversimplify. Part of knowing your audience is knowing their baseline understanding on the topic. Go too simple and you may offend rather than connect.

RESPOND IN THE MOMENT

When communicating, it's important to gauge the reactions of the people involved to ensure the message is getting through. Are they bored? Change the pace. Are they confused? State it in a different way. Are they angry? Stop and ask what's happening. Are they too quiet? Stop and get them more involved in what you are doing. Are they fidgeting, scribbling on their pads, or focusing on what's on their mobile device instead of your message? They may not be interested in what you are saying. Move to the end of your presentation or message. Check in with your audience frequently and select a different tactic if necessary.

 While course correcting in response to the audience's needs is critical to communicating, it's also important not to lose sight of your core message. Overcorrecting may send a signal that you lack conviction and your message could get lost altogether.

UNLEASH THE POWER OF QUESTIONS

Questions are a valuable tool—both for the person conveying the message and for those on the receiving end. Good communicators ask questions to get to a good understanding of their audience. On the flip side, questions you get tell you something about the audience and how successful you are being. When addressing a question, make sure you know what the question is. Ask one clarifying question before you answer: "Do you mean how would this product work in a foreign or domestic market?" Engage the audience when you can. Say "I have one way of thinking about that, but I'd like to hear what others think." Questions that challenge your message tell you that the person is trying to reconcile your message with his/her established mental model on the topic. Questions that expand on your message show that the person is trying to process your idea. Whatever the tone or content, questions equal engagement, which is always preferable to your being a talking head.

RESOURCES TO LEARN MORE

Gallo, C. (2009, March 24). Presentation lessons you didn't learn in B-school. *Bloomberg Businessweek.*

Sobel, A., & Panas, J. (2012). *Power questions: Build relationships, win new business, and influence others.* Hoboken, NJ: John Wiley & Sons.

Need to expand on the basics?
Master some communication mechanics.

BUILD MESSAGE STRUCTURE

State your message, intention, or purpose in a single sentence (or two), if possible. In other words, do the ending first. Then outline your talk around three to five things that support this thesis and that you want people to remember. More than that and the audience won't follow it. Say something like "There are three things I want you to remember. First…" You're likely to see people pull out their pens and take notice. Consider what an audience member should say 15 minutes after you finish. Use visual aids but don't overrely on them. When thinking about the length of your message, don't assume longer equals better. For speeches longer than 20 minutes, divide it into sections with clear conclusions and a hard bridge to the next related topic.

TELL A GOOD STORY

Even in today's hyper-technological world, stories remain a powerful means of communication. Why? Stories help us understand the world. Research has shown that young children use stories to understand cause and effect and to simplify the complex. When crafting your message, think about how to weave in storytelling. What will grab the audience and rivet them on your message? The best stories start strong and offer vivid images that can be easily remembered. They can center on a person, an event, or both. When the story you use is a personal one, you get the power of the story itself and also demonstrate authenticity to your audience. Tease out points from the story that reinforce your message. Find a key phrase that can be repeated. Refer back to those points throughout. It's likely that the key phrase will become a metaphor to help the audience find the meaning in your message.

POLISH YOUR TECHNIQUE

Like it or not, technique plays an important role in getting your message across. Use common action words, simple examples, or visual catchphrases to cement information transfer. Vary your volume and tone—sameness lulls the audience. Use pauses—for effect, to drive in a point. Be careful of repeating the same words too often. Avoid speaking too forcefully or using loaded terms that will annoy some audience members. If you're stumped for something to say, pause—uhs, ahs, and you knows distract and turn off some listeners. Draw a blank in the middle of your message? Pause, then repeat your last statement in a paraphrasing of it. While you play for time, ask yourself what you can connect to that statement. Rehearsing beforehand helps. Getting at ease with the content and technique of your message will free you up to scan the audience and adjust as you go.

15

RESOURCES TO LEARN MORE

Booth, D., Shames, D., & Desberg, P. (2010). *Own the room: Business presentations that persuade, engage, and get results.* New York, NY: McGraw-Hill.

Presentations Magazine. www.presentations.com

Simon, S. (2009, June 12). How to tell a story. National Public Radio Weekend Edition.

ASSIGNMENTS TO PRACTICE SKILL

Handle a tough negotiation with an external or internal customer to practice communicating outside-in, picking up on cues, and course correcting as needed.

Volunteer to craft and communicate a message across different cultural groups. Eastern cultures prefer lecture, Westerners prefer interactivity. Find ways to adapt your core message and delivery to fit different audience needs.

Be the spokesperson for an initiative that's important to you. Use storytelling to paint the picture for others of the value of what you propose.

TAKE TIME TO REFLECT...

Here are some questions to reflect on as you focus on being an Agile Communicator. Think about how you might answer these today and how, through using the tips in this chapter, you might achieve a better result in the future.

How often do you find yourself more concerned with demonstrating your expertise than getting a message across in a way that all can understand?

What are you doing to ensure that others understand the messages you'd like them to remember?

How do you differentiate the most important ideas for others?
When you speak, how often do you use industry or professional terminology?
How well does this translate to all of your audiences?

The single biggest problem in communication is the illusion that it has taken place.

George Bernard Shaw
Irish essayist, playwright, and literary critic

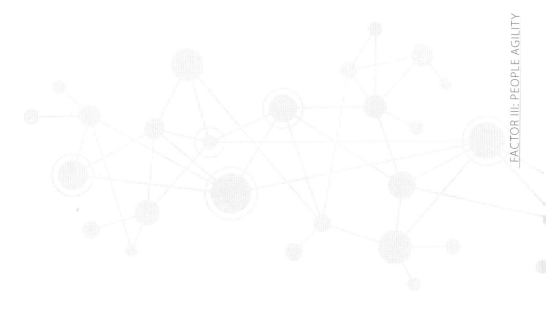

15

Conflict
Manager

Conflict is inevitable. Teams, organizations, and communities that are made up of diverse people with differing opinions and competing interests are primed for conflict. But conflict isn't necessarily a bad thing. Conflict can be revealing. Conflict highlights the intersection of ideas, provides an opportunity for finding better alternatives, and sharpens our thinking. But even more importantly, conflict provides an opportunity for breakthroughs, for changing hearts and minds, for building relationships and alliances. But only when the people involved treat each other constructively and respectfully. Otherwise, conflict can entrench. It can harden people's positions, sour them on relationships, and make them retreat behind their steadfast opinions. When you manage conflict effectively, you begin to see conflict as an opportunity. Then you do not shy away from it, but you also take care not to escalate it. Layers of unwavering convictions, strong feelings, and grievances do not deter you from engaging. Instead, you make sense of the tangle by seeing the issue from all sides and helping the parties involved see things from a more objective perspective. You are most effective when you manage conflict in the positive spirit of collaboration, mutual gain, and solution orientation.

A conflict begins and ends in the hearts and minds of people,
not in the hilltops.

Amos Oz
Israeli writer, novelist, and journalist

SKILLED

Stays positive, constructive, and respectful, even in disagreements or conflicts

Sees conflicts as opportunities for breakthroughs

Calmly negotiates resolutions and settles disputes

Defuses high-tension situations effectively

Finds common ground and win/win solutions

Open to changing his/her mind or position

LESS SKILLED

Avoids conflict

Is steadfast in his/her position on issues

Puts people on the defensive

Prioritizes own interests over others

Doesn't gauge impact on others well

OVERUSE OF SKILL

May take too long to reach a resolution

Overemphasizes consensus at the expense of reaching the best solution

Too eager to engage others in debate

Pushes for resolution before others are ready

SOME POSSIBLE CAUSES OF LOWER SKILL

Causes help explain "why" a person may have trouble in this dimension. When seeking to increase skill, it's helpful to consider how these might play out in certain situations. And remember that all of these can be addressed if you are motivated to do so.

Defensive

Doesn't listen

Gets stressed and frustrated easily

Has strong viewpoints on everything

Holds grudges

Impatient

Inflexible or rigid

Not observant

Strong need to dominate

Wants to win at all costs

Afraid to hurt others

DEVELOPMENTAL DIFFICULTY

When compared with other dimensions of Learning Agility, this dimension is **harder** to develop.

16

⭐ **Does It Best**

In 2007, Nelson Mandela formally launched The Elders, a group of global elders who no longer hold public office but represent the interests of global citizens as peacemakers. Members include Martti Ahtisaari, Kofi Annan, Ela Bhatt, Lakhdar Brahimi, Gro Harlem Brundtland, Fernando Cardoso, Jimmy Carter, Graca Machel, Mary Robinson, and Desmond Tutu. They work to mediate and resolve conflicts around the world, often in places where the situation seems beyond repair. Two of their guiding principles are maintaining an independent voice "not bound by the interests of any nation, government, or institution" and listening to everyone "no matter how unpalatable or unpopular this may be."[15] These are leaders whose experience and wisdom help them bring people together, foster dialogue, and find a path out of conflict and toward peaceful resolution.

TIPS TO INCREASE SKILL AS A CONFLICT MANAGER

Emotions running high?
Manage yourself to better manage conflict.

OVERCOME YOUR AVERSION TO CONFLICT

When emotions get triggered, many of us try to stay composed and in control by avoiding conflict altogether. By knowing what's happening in your brain and in your body, you can consciously work to counteract the tendency to duck and cover. Research shows that our brains perceive the threat of conflict as a threat to our status. And, according to our brains, maintaining or improving our status is of paramount importance because it ensures our survival. When our status is threatened, our limbic system is activated. More cortisol pumps through our body, anxiety increases, and we go into fight or flight mode. Awareness of this biological process can help you talk yourself down from the ledge and build up the courage to have a difficult conversation.

WATCH FOR TRIGGERS

Most of us have certain things that trigger us or set us off. What pushes your buttons? Do specific people, issues, styles, or groups set you off and make you handle the conflict poorly? Think about the last several times when you handled conflict poorly. What was common in the situations? Are there three to five common themes? Are the same people involved? Different people but the same style? Certain kinds of issues? Once you have isolated the cause, mentally rehearse a better way of handling it when it comes up next time.

FACTOR III: PEOPLE AGILITY

CHOOSE YOUR WORDS CAREFULLY

Words are powerful. Language, words, and timing set the tone and can cause unnecessary conflict that has to be managed before you can get anything done. Do you use insensitive language? Do you raise your voice often? Do you use terms and phrases that challenge others? Do you use demeaning terms? Do you use negative humor? Pick words that are other-person neutral. Pick words that don't challenge or sound one-sided. Pick tentative words that give others a chance to maneuver and save face. Pick words that are about the problem and not the person. Avoid direct blaming remarks; focus on the problem and its impact. Avoid global generalizations like "We have trust issues." To this respond, "Tell me your specific concern—why exactly don't you trust us, can you give me an example?" Keep the problem specific to the immediate situation.

RESOURCES TO LEARN MORE

Rock, D. (2009). *Your brain at work: Strategies for overcoming distraction, regaining focus, and working smarter all day long.* New York: NY: HarperCollins Publishers.

Winfrey, O. (2001, April). Oprah talks to Nelson Mandela [Interview]. *O, The Oprah Magazine.*

Tension escalating?
De-escalate the conflict.

SLOW DOWN

Conflict can be stressful and many people want it over with as quickly as possible. Impatient people provide solutions too early in the process. Take time to really define the problem and hear people out. Figure out what questions need to be answered in order to resolve it. Do you offer conclusions, solutions, statements, dictates, or answers early in the interaction? Give reasons first, solutions last. When you give solutions first, people often directly challenge the solutions instead of defining the problem and working toward a solution together.

 It is not always necessary to dwell on every point of disagreement. Balance listening with the decisive action when necessary. Putting consensus and harmony above all else can slow productivity down to a crawl.

OBSERVE WHAT'S GOING ON WITH OTHER PEOPLE

Rather than judging, focus on observing. People can sense your judgment, your disdain, your lack of interest. If you can't stay neutral and constructive, it's hard to expect other people to be solution oriented. Instead, observe and stay in tune with what others are experiencing and how they are reacting. If they are confused, state your argument differently. Angry? Stop and find out what's

16

going on. Too quiet? Ask a question, get them engaged. Disinterested? Figure out what's in it for them. Watch the reactions of people to what you are doing or saying. Be ready to adjust.

TURN AROUND TENSE INTERACTIONS

What if you're attacked? Let the other side vent frustration, blow off steam, but don't react directly. Remember that it's the person who hits back who usually gets in the most trouble. Listen. Nod. Ask clarifying questions. Ask open-ended questions like "Why is this particularly bothersome to you?" "What could I do to help?" "So you think I need to…." Restate the person's position periodically to signal you have understood. But don't react. Don't judge. Keep the person talking until he/she runs out of venom. When the other side takes a rigid position, don't reject it. Ask why—what's behind the position, what's the theory of the case, what brought this about? People will usually respond by saying more, coming off their position a bit, or at least revealing their true interests. Many times, with unlimited venting and your understanding, the actual conflict shrinks.

RESOURCES TO LEARN MORE

Flaxington, B. (2010). *Understanding other people: The five secrets to human behavior* (2nd ed.). ATA Press.

Trout, J. D. (2010). *Why empathy matters: The science and psychology of better judgment.* London, England: Penguin Books Ltd.

Want to see progress?
Work toward resolution.

SEEK OPPORTUNITIES TO BARGAIN OR TRADE

Each possesses something the other wants? Give in order to get. Seek opportunities to bargain and trade. Since you can't absolutely win all conflicts unless you keep pulling rank, you have to learn to trade and bargain. What do they need that I have? What could I do for them outside this conflict that could allow them to give up something I need now in return? How can we turn this into a win for both of us?

FIND COMMON GROUND

Almost all conflicts have common points that get lost in the heat of the battle. After a conflict has been presented and understood, start by saying that it might be helpful to see if we agree on anything. If it is difficult to find any overlapping interests, go to the most foundational common principles like "We both want this program to succeed," or "We all care about doing what's right for our customers and shareholders." Acknowledging this common ground serves to humanize all involved in the conflict. Focus on common goals, priorities, and problems. If you can't agree on a solution, agree on a procedure to move forward. Collect more data. Appeal to a higher power. Get a third-party arbitrator. Something. This creates some positive motion and breaks stalemates.

BE OPEN TO CHANGING YOUR MIND

In framing the disagreement, take the opportunity to state your position and explain your thinking. But when it comes to finding solutions, generate a variety of possibilities rather than staking out a rigid position. Stay open to possibilities you hadn't considered. The dialogue may surface opposing rationale, counterevidence, or ideas that you had not considered. Engaging in disagreements or conflicts where you show your willingness to change your mind is not a point of weakness, it's part of being a reasonable, level-headed person. Your willingness to concede on certain things builds a climate of cooperation and trust. And cooperative relationships are less likely to experience stalemate.

RESOURCES TO LEARN MORE

Levine, S. (2009). *Getting to resolution: Turning conflict into collaboration* (2nd ed.). San Francisco, CA: Berrett-Koehler Publishers.

Polsky, L., & Gerschel, A. (2011). *Perfect phrases for conflict resolution: Hundreds of ready-to-use phrases for encouraging a more productive and efficient work environment.* New York, NY: McGraw Hill.

ASSIGNMENTS TO PRACTICE SKILL

Make peace with an enemy or someone you've disappointed or someone you've had some trouble with or don't get along with. Apologize for your part in the conflict. Practice listening and find a solution that works for the greater good.

Resolve a conflict between two people or two departments. Get clear on the values and positions of each individual and gauge how that will play out during resolution efforts.

Assemble a team of diverse people to accomplish a difficult task. Anticipate the natural conflicts of ideas, interests, and personal styles this will bring about. Prepare to deepen team relationships by working through, rather than avoiding, conflict.

16

TAKE TIME TO REFLECT...

Here are some questions to reflect on as you focus on being a Conflict Manager. Think about how you might answer these today and how, through using the tips in this chapter, you might achieve a better result in the future.

Where have you seen conflict used in a healthy and advantageous way within a team? What did the team members do specifically that allowed conflict to be explored without destroying the team's effectiveness?

When have you avoided a conflict? Did it go away or did it fester? What were some of the benefits and drawbacks to skirting the issue? What would you do differently?

Think about a time when you had a breakthrough in a conflict or disagreement that you initially thought was unresolvable. What happened? What was instrumental to the breakthrough?

16

....

Conflict is inevitable in a team...in fact, to achieve synergistic solutions, a variety of ideas and approaches are needed. These are the ingredients for conflict.

Susan Gerke
American management consultant

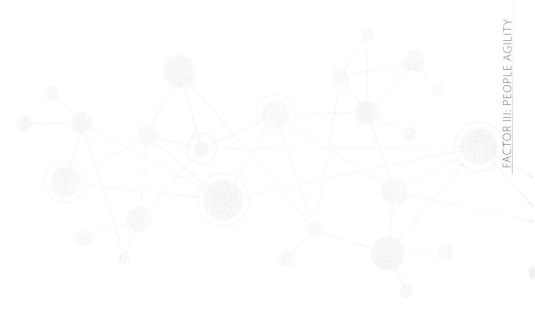

Helps
Others Succeed

Whether you are motivated by pure altruism or whether you know there's something in it for you, helping others succeed is in everyone's best interests. When you make your boss look good, that doesn't go unnoticed. When you share credit with your team members, they are more likely to recognize your contributions too. When you delegate, others can take on your old responsibilities so you can move on to something new. When you develop others, you raise everyone's game. The reality is that there is a limited amount any of us can accomplish on our own, regardless of how hard we work. Most people recognize this, but delegation and developing others continue to show up among the lowest leadership skills in all regions of the world. Even with the best intentions, either we don't know how to best help others succeed, or we are letting something else get in the way.

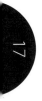

No man will make a great leader who wants to do it all himself,
or to get all the credit for doing it.

Andrew Carnegie
Scottish-born American industrialist and philanthropist

SKILLED

Steps aside and lets others shine

Likes to see others do well

Is available as a mentor and coach

Helps others apply their strengths and shore up their weaknesses

Provides the right amount of challenge and autonomy

LESS SKILLED

Is unaware of people's needs

Delegates too much or too little

Prefers to work alone;
too self-sufficient

Struggles to share credit

Envies the success of others

Takes a more competitive than
collaborative approach

Sees success as a zero-sum game

Assumes that success means
the same thing to everyone

OVERUSE OF SKILL

Is overly optimistic about how much
people can grow

Gives up too much responsibility
and accountability

May overdelegate

Creates a false sense of
accomplishment in others

SOME POSSIBLE CAUSES OF LOWER SKILL

Causes help explain "why" a person may have trouble in this dimension. When seeking to increase skill, it's helpful to consider how these might play out in certain situations. And remember that all of these can be addressed if you are motivated to do so.

Works alone	Jealous of others
Doesn't take the time	Selfish
Excessively high standards	Short-term perspective
Fears failure	Too competitive
Grandstands	Unappreciative

DEVELOPMENTAL DIFFICULTY

When compared with other dimensions of Learning Agility, this dimension is **_easier_** to develop.

159

17

🔎 Did You Know?

Many managers are under the misconception that people are primarily motivated by money and title. In actuality, there are many more things that rise to the top of people's lists. According to research by Renwick and Lawler,[16] the top motivators at work are (1) job challenge, (2) accomplishing something worthwhile, (3) learning new things, (4) personal development, and (5) autonomy. Other motivators, including pay (12th), friendliness (14th), praise (15th), or chance of promotion (17th), are not insignificant but are superficial compared with the more powerful motivators. Don't bet on the wrong motivators. Provide challenges, paint pictures of why this is worthwhile, create a common mind-set, set up chances to learn and grow, and provide autonomy, and you'll hit the vast majority of people's hot buttons.

TIPS TO INCREASE SKILL IN HELPS OTHERS SUCCEED

Looking to make a difference?
Mentor, teach, develop others.

UNDERSTAND THE STARTING POINT

Do you have a sense of the individual's current state? Size up a person's skill profile with an informal appraisal. You can't help anyone develop if you can't or aren't willing to fairly and accurately appraise people. Sound appraisal starts with the best picture of current strengths and weaknesses. Then you need to know what competencies are going to be necessary going forward. Unless you know where the person is and where they need to go, it's difficult to chart a course to get there.

TAILOR YOUR EFFORT TO UNIQUE NEEDS

Developing others is not a one-size-fits-all proposition. People have different backgrounds, levels of experience, learning styles, and preferences. Make sure you know who you are working with before you rely on what worked for someone else. Taking a more flexible approach can mean slowing down or speeding up, having more patience or more urgency, providing more or less direction, a different tone, and different rewards and encouragement. Be sure to check in and get feedback on how you are doing and what you can do better. After all, coaching and mentoring are skills, and you are developing yourself even as you develop others.

FIND STRETCHING ASSIGNMENTS

As a people developer, one of your roles is to act as a broker between people and assignments. When you know a person's strengths and weaknesses as well as their areas of interest, you are uniquely poised to play matchmaker. Find progressively stretching tasks that are first-time and different for each person. At least 70% of reported development occurs through challenging assignments that demand skill development. People don't grow from doing more of the same. Encourage them to think of themselves as learners, not just accomplishers. Help them process what they are learning from tough assignments. What are they learning that is new or different? What skills have improved in the last year? What have they learned that they can use in other situations?

> **RESOURCES TO LEARN MORE**
>
> Flaherty, J. (2010). *Coaching: Evoking excellence in others* (3rd ed.). Oxford, England: Butterworth-Heinemann.
>
> Orr, J. E. (2012). *Becoming an agile leader: A guide to learning from your experiences.* Minneapolis, MN: Lominger International: A Korn/Ferry Company.

Trying to be a hero?
Delegate more.

MATCH THE RIGHT FEAT TO THE RIGHT PERSON

Get comfortable handing over control to others. You've assembled a talented team; let them shine. All of your people have differing skills and capacities. Good delegators match the size and complexity of the delegated task with the capacity of each person. Delegation is not an equal, one-size-fits-all, activity. Equal opportunity delegators are not as successful as equitable delegators. Most people prefer stretching tasks to those they could do in their sleep; so it's OK to give each person a task slightly bigger than his/her current capabilities might dictate. Engage each person in the sizing task. Ask them. Most will select wisely.

 Take care not to let the pendulum swing too far. Hoarding work is no good, but overdelegating is not much better. If you overdelegate, you are putting a heavy burden on your team, and they may not feel set up for success.

SET CLEAR EXPECTATIONS

State your expectations, share the information you know, then get out of the way. One of the most common problems with delegation is incomplete or cryptic up-front communication leading to frustration, a job not well done the first time, rework, and a reluctance to delegate next time. When you've been clear about your expectations, you can let out some slack. Let other people take accountability for the work, follow up, and offer help as needed. It's a

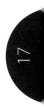

good idea to adjust your own expectations too. Other people may take longer and may approach the job differently and they may need different support. That's all part of the work of helping people be successful.

COMMUNICATE THE *WHAT* AND THE *WHY*, LET THEM DETERMINE THE *HOW*
Explain why the work is important. Although it is not necessary to get the task done, people are more motivated when they know where it fits in the bigger picture. And be very clear on what and when. Provide the right amount of detail. What does the outcome look like? When do you need it by? What's the budget? What resources do they get? What decisions can they make? Do you want checkpoints along the way? How will we both know and measure how well the task is done? Then, resist micromanaging. Be very open on how the thing gets done. Inexperienced delegators include the hows, which turn people into task automatons instead of an empowered and energized staff. People are more motivated when they can determine the how themselves. Encourage them to try things. Besides being more motivating, it's also more developmental for them.

> **RESOURCES TO LEARN MORE**
> Garner, E. (2012). *Delegation and empowerment: Giving people the chance to excel* [eBook version].
> Spiro, J. (2010, April 16). How to delegate properly. *Inc.com*

Want others to rise to the occasion?
Motivate people to be their best.

SET PEOPLE UP FOR SUCCESS BY SHARING WHAT YOU KNOW
It's not motivating for people when they miss out on details and information that could help them do a better job. Think about how well you keep your team informed. Do you hold back information? Do you parcel out information on your schedule? Do you share information to get an advantage or to win favor? Do people around you know what you're doing and why? Are you aware of things others would benefit from but you don't take the time to communicate? Organizations and teams function on the flow of information. Make sure that you're not the impediment.

FACTOR III: PEOPLE AGILITY

ENCOURAGE PEOPLE TO TAKE ON A CHALLENGE

Part of developing others is convincing people that tough, new, challenging, and different assignments are good for them. In follow-up studies of successful executives, more than 90% report that a boss in their past nearly forced them to take a scary job assignment they wanted to turn down. That assignment turned out to be the most developmental for them. The peculiar thing about long-term development is that even ambitious people turn down the very assignments they need to grow. They do not have the perspective to understand that. Your job is to help convince people on the way up to get out of their comfort zone and accept jobs they don't initially see as useful or leading anywhere.

LET OTHERS SHINE

Somewhere along the way, someone brought out the best in you. Think about how you can do that for others around you. Tone down your competitiveness long enough to give credit where it is due. Take time to recognize and celebrate success. Be an advocate and a champion for the people you believe in. Make it part of your role and legacy to help others flourish in their careers. In the long run, you will cultivate many grateful fans and a favorable reputation as someone who can spot and develop top talent.

> **RESOURCES TO LEARN MORE**
> Basheer, T. (2008). 10 Ways to be a good mentor. Blue Sky Coaching.
> Pink, D. (2009, August 25). The puzzle of motivation [Video file].

ASSIGNMENTS TO PRACTICE SKILL

Manage a group of people where you are the towering expert and they are beginners. Help them with a task they could not do by themselves. Gradually build their independence and confidence.

Manage a team fixing something that has failed, where the same team who failed will stay to get it right. Help them succeed and let them take credit for the success.

Manage a group of people in a rapidly expanding unit that has to learn new things quickly. Help them develop the skills they need. Delegate responsibility to build skill and confidence.

TAKE TIME TO REFLECT...

Here are some questions to reflect on as you focus on Helps Others Succeed. Think about how you might answer these today and how, through using the tips in this chapter, you might achieve a better result in the future.

How do you ensure that people on a team are recognized for their contributions? What do you do to help make the team operate effectively? Where might you be detracting from teamwork?

Where might people in your organization lack clarity on how their jobs directly contribute to the organization's success? What are you doing to ensure that others understand how their roles contribute to the success of the organization?

Think back to a time where you were given a tremendous amount of responsibility before others might have felt you were ready for it or deserved it. Did anyone help you achieve success in that situation? Who? How did they help? How can you create similar experiences in others?

17

....

Few things help an individual more than to place responsibility upon him, and to let him know that you trust him.

Booker T. Washington
American educator, author, orator, and political leader

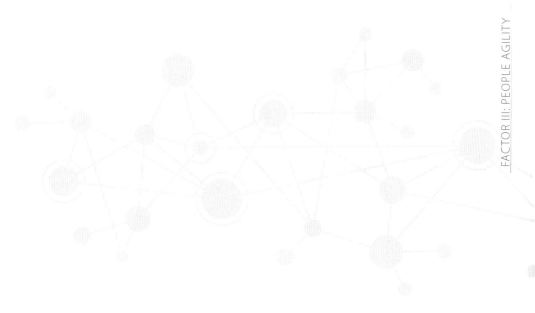

17

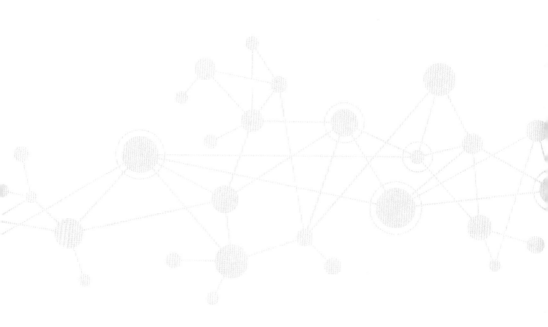

Change Agility

Change Agility means viewing established ways of doing things with a questioning eye, recognizing that in today's hyper-volatile and complex world, status quo too often signals decline or even extinction for organizations. A change agile person sees opportunities to continuously improve everywhere—from the day-to-day to the transformational. They pose the big questions: What if…? Why? Why not? This makes them idea magnets, open to even the most seemingly far-fetched suggestions for solving unmet customer needs or future problems. With their ability to anticipate future consequences and trends accurately, they will usually introduce a new way of viewing a problem or opportunity. And their default is to give something a try, even when some things may still be undefined. Because they see trial and error as a proxy for learning, someone high in Change Agility does not see mistakes as failures. To the contrary—for them, *not* trying equals failure. And as much as the change agile person thrives on experimenting with new things, they also recognize that the world is littered with great ideas that no one was able to figure out how to implement. Or that died a slow, painful death mired in organizational politics. The change agile person recognizes which ideas are the best bets to take to market and can navigate through formal and informal channels to manage an idea through to implementation. Understanding that being on the forefront of change can be a lonely and unpopular place to be, someone high in Change Agility balances objectivity and empathy in managing others' discomfort with change.

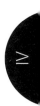

DIMENSIONS

Continuous Improver

Visioning

Experimenter

Innovation Manager

Comfort Leading Change

Continuous
Improver

The world we operate in today is one where complexity is up and certainty is down. Where more and more often, conventional wisdom seems to be losing its surety. Where growth is now far from a given for companies. In this environment, reinventing yourself is no longer a guarantee that you (or your organization) will thrive—it isn't a "one time and you're set" proposition. Success hinges on constantly improving—so you're never done, never satisfied, never standing in place. Continuously improving is about much more than processes. It's a mind-set. A mind-set that views established ways of doing things with a questioning eye: Can we make this better? Why do it this way? What would happen if we tried…? Being a Continuous Improver means that you retain a healthy dose of skepticism about the current state of things. And that you find golden nuggets where you can innovate and change fast, in both small and big ways. In a reality where status quo has become the equivalent to moving backward, continuously improving puts you steps ahead and keeps you moving forward.

You are doing your best only when you are trying to improve
what you are doing.

Author Unknown

SKILLED

Operates from the mind-set that "as is" should always be questioned

Is never satisfied with the status quo

Sees opportunity to innovate in both the small stuff and the big stuff

Constantly evaluates existing processes, procedures, and ways of doing things

Can't leave things alone for long without seeking a new way

LESS SKILLED

Protects traditional ways of getting things done

Avoids disturbances to existing processes and methods

Doesn't examine things that seem to be working

Prefers work that is orderly and routine

Likes it when things are settled

OVERUSE OF SKILL

May undervalue proven methods and processes

Doesn't pause to allow what's been improved to take root

Is scattered; can't prioritize the things that truly need improving

Obsessed with changing things

SOME POSSIBLE CAUSES OF LOWER SKILL

Causes help explain "why" a person may have trouble in this dimension. When seeking to increase skill, it's helpful to consider how these might play out in certain situations. And remember that all of these can be addressed if you are motivated to do so.

Dislikes the noise of change

Fears failing in the new

Fears uncertainty

Gets stressed and anxious easily

Not curious

Prefers predictability

Too comfortable

Clings to the past

Low risk orientation

DEVELOPMENTAL DIFFICULTY

When compared with other dimensions of Learning Agility, this dimension is **_easier_** to develop.

18

Did You Know?

In a recent interview with *Fast Company* magazine, Beth Comstock, chief marketing officer of global powerhouse General Electric, talked about the imperative of continuous reinvention: "Business-model innovation is constant in this economy. You start with a vision of a platform. For a while, you think there's a line of sight, and then it's gone. There's suddenly a new angle. We need to systematize change."[17]

TIPS TO INCREASE SKILL AS A CONTINUOUS IMPROVER

Have a bias for "as is"?
Rewire yourself.

OVERRIDE YOUR DEFAULT COMFORT MODE

If you find yourself defaulting to the established way of doing things, you're not alone. It turns out our brains are conditioned to be more comfortable with the status quo. We have a natural tendency to stick to what is already known, what we've already decided, what's comfortable. Change of any kind makes our brains work harder than staying the same does. The good news is that we can override our brain's natural tendency toward inertia. How? By constantly trying something new—new ways of doing things, new experiences, new people. There will be "switching costs" for you at first. You're bound to feel a decreased sense of mastery and will likely fail sometimes too. By focusing on the payoff—being able to more easily adapt and even being out in front on change—you can silence that worry voice inside your head that keeps you tethered to what's comfortable and familiar.

KICK THE HABIT HABIT

One way to get out of your routine way of thinking is to get out of your routine. If you find yourself with a short list of favorite things, it's probably past time to expose yourself more to the unfamiliar. Attend perspective-broadening lectures and workshops on topics that you normally don't attend. Go to the theater, concerts, and other cultures' festivals. Travel to and vacation in different locales. Change up day-to-day things—drive to work a different way, use the computer mouse with your opposite hand, rearrange how the apps on your mobile devices are organized. Stimulate your brain by doing things, going places, and talking to people outside of your routine. To stay in constant innovation mode, constantly ask yourself is there anything new to learn here? Anything that may surprise me? Remember that, though it may feel uncomfortable at first, the more newness you weave into your life, the more of a habit it will become in itself.

MANAGE STRESS

When you're under pressure or stress, it's harder to step away from what's comfortable. In stress mode, we go to habits more readily, which stops us from taking new actions. Why? For us to be able to integrate new information properly, things have to be relatively quiet in the brain. In the research on executive derailment, making decisions under intense pressure often led the executives to preemptively land (incorrectly) on a favorite past solution. Find ways to manage your stress levels. Give your mind clear and repetitious breakpoints—for instance, between work and non-work stressors. Signal work is over by playing music in your car (try a new station every day—remember, embedding newness wherever you can works that adaptability muscle), immediately play with your kids, go for a walk, swim for 20 minutes. At work, worry about work things, not life things. When you hit the driveway, worry about life things and leave work things at the office.

RESOURCES TO LEARN MORE

Bloomberg Businessweek. (2008, December 4). Managing stress can improve company performance. *Bloomberg Businessweek*.

Cutts, M. (2011, July). Try something new for 30 days [Video file].

Think the only way to change is large-scale?
Go small to go big.

USE YOUR COMPANY AS YOUR CLASSROOM

Whether it's the next big idea or a hundred smaller ones that lead to continuous improvement, having a deep, solid understanding of your business is a must. So become a student of your business. Reduce your understanding of how business operates to personal rules of thumb or insights. Write them down in your own words. An example would be "What are the drivers in marketing anything?" One executive had 25 such drivers that he continuously edited, scratched through, and replaced with more up-to-date ones. Another helpful route is to talk to the people who know. Meet with strategic partners and key customers. Read about your business and industry in the press. Get to know your competitors and your customers' competitors. With this increased understanding, it will be easier to visualize initiatives that could make a huge difference.

18

FIND A REAL-LIFE LABORATORY TO PILOT IMPROVEMENT

Be a pilot for a change that can eventually come to life organizationwide. In a four-year study of corporate change, it wasn't the big processes, structural changes, or programs, but the ad hoc, business-problem-focused stuff in the business (often on the periphery) that infused new ways of thinking into the organization. In those instances and in the best way, infection took hold. The pioneer institution in the microlending movement, Grameen Bank, started as a university project where money was loaned without collateral to a group of village stool makers. So don't think that starting small means you're not willing to risk. By choosing a relatively safe environment at first, it will help keep your brain's risk-averse triggers at bay. Start small, and repeat in ever-increasing scope. This way, you will always be moving forward, constantly improving.

TAKE CALCULATED RISKS

Almost by definition, continuously improving involves pushing the envelope, taking chances, and trying out something that is untested. Doing these things will inevitably lead to more misfires and mistakes in the short-term but will ultimately yield better results. Start to treat any mistakes or failures as chances to learn. Nothing ventured, nothing gained. Remember that most successful innovations are usually the result of multiple trials and errors. American inventor Thomas Edison always viewed failures in the lab as mini-successes. In his view, each time an attempt didn't work, it got him closer to the solution that would.

> **RESOURCES TO LEARN MORE**
> Branson, R. (2010, November 1). The art of calculated risk. *Entrepreneur*.
> Kaplan, R., & Mikes, A. (2012). Managing risks: A new framework. *Harvard Business Review, 90*(6), 48–60.

Think you need to go it alone?
Be an improvement magnet.

PREPARE YOUR CASE AND PRESENT IT WITH STRENGTH

Do your homework. Be prepared. Don't make it sound like a trial balloon. Use more definite, direct language. Don't be vague or tentative. Don't throw things out without the air cover of the business case and the safety net of how everybody can gain by the improvement you propose. Prepare by rehearsing for tough questions, attacks, and countering views. Plan as if you're only going to have one shot. Match your style, tone, pace, and volume with the feeling that you are right and that this thing must get done. Lead with strength.

Don't underestimate the extent of others' trepidation about change. If you ram through your ideas without due consideration of people's feelings and concerns, you may win in the short-term, but you will do so at the expense of relationships with the very people you need to sustain the change.

BRING OTHERS ALONG WITH YOU

For any meaningful and sustained improvements to take hold, you can't go it alone. You can be the champion, but not alone on the field. It's important to establish a sense of urgency in the people you need to execute and adopt changes you propose. In this way, you create a pull rather than a push—people will feel a sense of ownership, that they're part of the solution. Having people live with the problem themselves helps. The former head of the New York Transit Police required officers to commute by subway so they could witness firsthand the need for increased security. Now New York City subways have a much stronger image and record of safety.

GET THE NAYSAYERS ONBOARD

When you try new ways of doing things, people will always say it should have been done differently. Listen to them, but be skeptical. Conduct a postmortem immediately after finishing. This will indicate to all that you're committed to continuous improvement, whether the result was stellar or not. If you have trouble going back a second or third time to get people onboard with your innovation, then switch approaches. For example, you could meet with all stakeholders, a single key stakeholder, present the idea to a group, call in an expert to buttress your innovation, or project various scenarios showing the value of the idea. Another tactic is to tap one of your critics for a key role on the team. Seeing a respected senior insider standing shoulder to shoulder with you will send a powerful message of support through the ranks.

RESOURCES TO LEARN MORE

Best, M. (2012, May 14). Get the corporate antibodies on your side. *Harvard Business Review*.

Crom, M. (2012, February 3). Answer tough questions with honesty, explanation. *USA Today*.

ASSIGNMENTS TO PRACTICE SKILL

Form an improvement-focused start-up in your own department or area. This will give you an opportunity to gain deep understanding of what's working and what's not working and what changes (small, medium, large) would help keep the department nimble and adaptable.

Relaunch an existing product or service that's not doing well by trying things not tried before. It's likely you will have some air cover to test out new ideas and methods since the conventional options obviously hadn't worked previously.

Work on a project that involves travel and study of an issue, acquisition, or joint venture in a part of the world that is unfamiliar to you, and report back to management. You will be exposed to many things that are unfamiliar and will need to use that new knowledge to inform your recommendations.

18

TAKE TIME TO REFLECT...

Here are some questions to reflect on as you focus on being a Continuous Improver. Think about how you might answer these today and how, through using the tips in this chapter, you might achieve a better result in the future.

In what areas do you strive for continuous improvement? What motivates you toward excellence? How will you hang on to this inspiration?

In your current role, who are your customers? How do your customers interfere with your job? What improvements could you introduce that would better serve both your customers and your ability to deliver value for them?

What potential do you see for solutions in the problems you currently face? How can you channel your focus from what is wrong or broken to how it can be improved? What is one specific area where you will begin to explore solutions?

Where might you feel stuck in a proverbial rut? What is one thing you can begin doing today to break the habit of sameness? How might doing something differently improve your satisfaction with the process or outcome?

A relentless barrage of "whys" is the best way to prepare your mind to pierce the clouded veil of thinking caused by the status quo. Use it often.

Shigeo Shingo
Japanese industrial engineer and one of the world's leading experts on manufacturing practices and the Toyota Production System

18

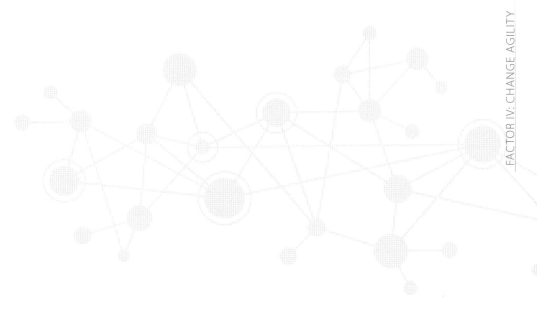

Visioning

Visioning the future doesn't come from fairy tales, fortune telling, or random creative thought, but as a result of careful study. The study of history and of trends that are starting to take shape. Of parallels and the lessons learned by others. How successful could you be if you could forecast which stocks will go up in the market? The next way to organize companies to be more productive? What about the next trend in your business? The next market or country to latch on to your product or service? The next big thing in your product line? Change leadership guru John Kotter describes these as windows of opportunity—ones that are coming at us faster all the time, yet staying open for shorter and shorter lengths of time. Visioning gives you the key to unlock those future-opportunity windows and increases your chances of acting on target when the future gets here. The best way to prepare for an event is to know about it ahead of time. An even better path is to create the future you want.

The future belongs to those who see possibilities
before they become obvious.

John Sculley
American businessman, former president of PepsiCo, and CEO of Apple Computer

19

SKILLED
Good at envisioning "what ifs"
Can anticipate future consequences and trends accurately
Introduces a new way of viewing a problem or opportunity
Sees ahead clearly
Can project multiple future scenarios
Articulately paints credible pictures of possibilities and likelihoods

LESS SKILLED

May have trouble seeing fresh scenarios or where they might lead

Has narrow view of issues and challenges

A here-and-now person who is often surprised by unexpected change

May be more comfortable with the past, prefers the tried and true

Uses old solutions for new problems

Prefers concrete solutions

OVERUSE OF SKILL

Isn't grounded in reality

Has difficulty deciding on the one best way to move forward

Dismisses conventional wisdom without due process

SOME POSSIBLE CAUSES OF LOWER SKILL

Causes help explain "why" a person may have trouble in this dimension. When seeking to increase skill, it's helpful to consider how these might play out in certain situations. And remember that all of these can be addressed if you are motivated to do so.

Avoids risks

Doesn't like being first or out front of others

Doesn't like to speculate

Fears rejection of ideas

Narrow background

Not creative

Not curious

Prefers past solutions

Prefers to stick with what is known

Short-term focus

DEVELOPMENTAL DIFFICULTY
When compared with other dimensions of Learning Agility, this dimension is **harder** to develop.

19

⭐ **Does It Best**

Half a century ago, Lee Kuan Yew, former Singaporean prime minister, often referred to as the father of modern Singapore, had a vision for what was possible in his country. Lee's "big idea" was that, in order for Singapore to realize its potential, the citizens would first need a prosperous livelihood and have a sense of nationalism. One thing Lee did immediately was to compel citizens to adopt English as their working language. This helped forge a unified society and laid the foundation to unite the island's many different ethnic groups. Lee wanted to instill in his fellow Singaporeans a sense that they all shared a future, in his words, that "if Singapore goes down everyone goes down."[18]

Through Lee's vision, Singapore has been transformed from a fishing village with a port to an intellectual and technical center of the region. Due in large part to his leadership, per capita income has grown from about $400 a year to close to $40,000, and what was a medium-sized city has become a significant international and economic player.

TIPS TO INCREASE SKILL IN VISIONING

Focused mostly on the tactical?
Flex your strategic muscles.

BE CURIOUS AND IMAGINATIVE

Many managers are so wrapped up in today's problems that they aren't curious about tomorrow. They really don't care about the long-term future. They may not even see themselves in the organization when the strategic plan is supposed to happen. They believe there won't be much of a future until *we perform today*. But too much emphasis on the short-term can leave you ill-prepared to anticipate future trends. Being a visionary and a good strategist requires curiosity and imagination. What are the implications of the growing gap between rich and poor? The collapse of retail pricing? The increasing influence of brand names? What will happen when a larger percentage of the world's population is over the age of 65? The effects of terrorism? What if cancer is cured? Heart disease? AIDS? Obesity? What if the government outlaws or severely regulates some aspect of your business? True, nobody knows the answers, but good strategists know the questions. Work

19

at developing broader interests outside your business. Subscribe to different magazines. Pick new shows to watch. Meet different people. Join a new organization. Look under some rocks. Think about tomorrow. Talk to others about what they think the future will bring.

The world is full of orphaned ideas that were never implemented because the person with the vision became so enamored of the idea process that execution was never considered. Know the right questions to ask to get ideas flowing, but also know when it's time to stop questioning and start acting.

PRACTICE STRATEGIC THINKING
Strategy is linking several variables together to come up with the most likely scenario. Think of it as the search for and application of relevant parallels. It involves making projections of several variables at once to see how they come together. These projections are in the context of shifting markets, international affairs, monetary movements, and government interventions. It involves a lot of uncertainty, making risk assumptions, and understanding how things work together. How many reasons would account for sales going down? Up? How are advertising and sales linked? If the dollar is cheaper in Asia, what does that mean for our product in that region? If the world population is aging and has more money, how will that change buying patterns?

RECOGNIZE THAT STRATEGY IS NO SYNONYM FOR CERTAINTY
Strategic planning is the most uncertain thing managers do, next to managing people. It's speculating on the near-unknown. It requires projections into foggy landscapes. It requires assumptions about the unknown. Many conflict avoiders and perfectionists don't like to make statements in public that they cannot back up with facts. Most strategies can be challenged and questioned. There are no clean ways to win a debate over strategy. It really comes down to one subjective estimate versus another. If you're questioned, think of this as a good thing. Questions from others are really opportunities to further vet your strategic direction, raise issues you may not have thought of, and likely yield a sounder approach as a result.

RESOURCES TO LEARN MORE
Kotter, J. P. (1996). *Leading change.* Boston, MA: Harvard Business School Press.

Watkins, M. (2007, April 20). How to think strategically. *Harvard Business Review.*

19

Tend to think in concrete terms?
Fill your "what if" funnel.

SEEK OUT A BROAD ARRAY OF SOURCES

Part of visioning involves asking a series of educated "what ifs" when trying to anticipate future scenarios. The more possibilities you can come up with, the closer you'll be to having a plan once the future arrives. To make more informed guesses, read periodicals with a global perspective, such as the *New York Times*, the *Economist*, *International Herald Tribune*, *Bloomberg Businessweek*, *Forbes,* and the *Atlantic*. These periodicals do an excellent job of setting historical context as well as explaining how things got to be the way they are. If you're stuck in the present, using history is also helpful to find parallels. There are always plenty of candidates. U.S. president Harry Truman used the presidential archives to form a "council of presidents" to see what his predecessors had done in parallel situations. The more you know about past and present trends, the better your "what ifs" will become.

USE FUTURE-FOCUSED PROJECTIONS AS A GUIDEPOST

Read *Management Challenges for the 21st Century* by Peter Drucker, any of the *Megatrends* books by John Naisbitt, the *Popcorn Report* by Faith Popcorn, economic growth forecasts from The Conference Board, or the *Futurist*, a journal of the World Future Society. For example, The Conference Board is predicting that economic growth between now and 2025 in developed countries will be 1%–3% annually. In developing countries, the estimate is 2%–6%. What will this slower growth mean to your business? Does this mean more of a focus on mitigating risk and less on not missing out on investment opportunities? In Drucker's book, he raises issues such as what does it mean that the birth rate is collapsing in the developed world? Will the retirement age go up? Will we treat workers more like volunteers as they opt out of larger organizations? The means of production has largely become knowledge. Is this a harbinger of more outsourcing and alliances? Or will protectionism begin to gain a stronger foothold? What are the trends at play and how do they affect your organization going forward?

CONNECT UNRELATED KNOWNS TO ENVISION THE NEW

Fresh ideas don't spontaneously spring forth from hydroponic ponds. They are planted and nurtured by your experiences and the experiences of those around you. More often, new ideas are a result of cross-pollinating those experiences—making fresh connections that lead to something new. Often, the greatest innovators came from a field adjacent to the one in which they had their breakthrough. Consider the modern minivan or people carrier which wasn't dreamed up out of thin air. It was a result of combining the cargo-hauling features of full-sized vans with the ride comfort and other consumer-friendly features of a station wagon.

RESOURCES TO LEARN MORE

Cope, K. (2012). *Seeing the big picture: Business acumen to build your credibility, career, and company.* Austin, TX: Greenleaf Book Group.

Ringland, G. (2006). *Scenario planning: Managing for the future* (2nd ed.). West Sussex, England: John Wiley & Sons Ltd.

Think visioning all happens in your own head?
Have a visioning game plan.

SEE THE LOGIC IN BEING ILLOGICAL

Many of us are driven by logic, but fresh ideas often come from a mind that is a bit sillier. You don't have to tell anyone what you're doing. Ask what song is this problem like? Find an analogy to your situation in nature, in children's toys, in anything that has a physical structure. Don't just focus on what makes sense or is intuitive when coming up with something new. Look for anomalies, unusual facts that don't quite fit in. Why did sales go down when they should have gone up? It could be random, but maybe not. Look for patterns, something present in failures but not present in successes. Even more useful, look for elements present in successes but never present in a failure. This will yield some insight into underlying principles.

WORK ON YOUR VISUAL SIDE

Concrete thinking is helpful when it's time to implement a big idea, but it can get in the way of coming up with that big idea in the first place. The good news is there are some concrete tools that can help nurture new ideas. One is storyboarding, a pictorial technique of representing a problem or process. Another is mind mapping, a wonderfully branching way to plan, examine ideas, and simply think differently. Get some scenario training, then implement it with your team to come up with likely futures. Use flowcharting software packages. Close your eyes and see what the outcome would look like. Come up with an image or symbol that embodies the vision. When it comes time to sell your vision to others, remember that people are much more likely to get excited by stories, symbols, and images than a white paper explaining the plan.

EXPAND YOUR PEOPLE RESOURCES

If you find yourself brainstorming the same ideas over and over again, expand the brain trust. Convene a group with the widest possible variety of backgrounds. (Yes, we mean widest. It makes no difference if they know

19

anything about the problem.) The design firm IDEO looks for T-shaped people when forming a creative team—people with a deep knowledge in a single area and a broad ability to relate in a broad collaborative process. You're looking for fresh approaches here, not practicality. That comes later as you sift through the ideas. Strategy-based scenario planning uses this technique as a best practice. At one multinational telecommunications company, scenario planning participants included a painter, a musician, and a prep school athletic coach in addition to company representatives and industry insiders.

RESOURCES TO LEARN MORE

Hansen, M. (2010, January 21). IDEO CEO Tim Brown: T-Shaped stars: The backbone of IDEO's collaborative culture. *Chief Executive.net.*

Kanter, R. M. (2011). How great companies think differently. *Harvard Business Review, 89*(11), 66-79.

ASSIGNMENTS TO PRACTICE SKILL

Prepare and present a strategic proposal of some consequence to top management which involves a change in direction and where newness will be a mandate.

Seek out and use a seed budget to create and pursue a personal idea, product, or service. Draw upon more than the "usual suspect" resources to help you visualize how your big idea can add value to your intended audience or customer.

Do a rotation in a company strategy position which requires significant strategic thinking and planning, charts new ground, and involves selling the vision to a critical audience.

19

TAKE TIME TO REFLECT...

Here are some questions to reflect on as you focus on Visioning. Think about how you might answer these today and how, through using the tips in this chapter, you might achieve a better result in the future.

How can you expand your views to what is possible and not just what is likely, based on current trends?

In brainstorming sessions, how often do you find yourself saying, "That won't work"? How many ideas may have been squashed by holes you may have inadvertently poked in them? What would happen if you let the idea generation unfold without intervening?

When have you seen the perfect balance between a vision and the action taken to reach it? How were the two intertwined? Why was it necessary for both to be present in order for vision to be realized?

....

I skate to where the puck is going to be, not where it has been.

Wayne Gretzky
Hall of Fame Canadian hockey player

19

Experimenter

So much of what we read about innovation centers on the outcome, the big finish, and less on the journey toward that outcome. But the truth is that most changes come as a result of a long road of trial and error, mistakes, even accidents. The more experiments, the more chances to learn to do something better. Too often, we do things the same old way, yet expect a different outcome. Trial and error eventually leads to improvement. Being an Experimenter means you are tirelessly trying, putting yourself out there, risking failure because you know that failure equals learning. Learning what not to do the next time you try. The household product WD-40® didn't get its name from market research or focus groups—it took 39 previous unsuccessful tries to finally get the water displacement (WD) formula right. It took Thomas Edison thousands of tries. Most of the things we use today in life were not created instantly. Instead, they came along as the very last car in a long experimenting train.

I have not failed.
I've just found 10,000 ways that won't work.

Thomas Edison
American inventor and businessman

20

SKILLED
Enjoys experimenting with test cases
Views failures as opportunities for learning
Comfortable trying several times before finding the right solution
Floats trial balloons
Tries products and services not quite ready
Sees mistakes as a necessary part of innovation process

LESS SKILLED
Likes to have everything just so

Is critical of imperfections inherent in experiments

Thinks experimentation equates to sloppiness

Holds changes up to impossibly mature standards

Tends to be skeptical of unproven ideas

Collects and analyzes lots of data to be sure of success

OVERUSE OF SKILL
Can't sense when it's time to quit

Doesn't consider possible collateral damage when experiments go awry

Undervalues orderly problem solving, analysis, and careful implementation

Takes unnecessary risks

SOME POSSIBLE CAUSES OF LOWER SKILL
Causes help explain "why" a person may have trouble in this dimension. When seeking to increase skill, it's helpful to consider how these might play out in certain situations. And remember that all of these can be addressed if you are motivated to do so.

Can't think of anything new or different

Comfortable with what is

Defensive

Doesn't like taking risks

Doesn't like to be out front leading

Fears failure and making mistakes

Impatient

Not curious

Perfectionist

DEVELOPMENTAL DIFFICULTY
When compared with other dimensions of Learning Agility, this dimension is ***moderately difficult*** to develop.

⭐ **Does It Best**

British entrepreneur and experimenter Sir James Dyson reports that he built 5,127 prototypes of his cyclonic vacuum before getting to one that was commercially successful. Though his vacuums are pricier than most, today Dyson enjoys what some reports cite as a 37% share of the vacuum cleaner market and continues to raise the bar on innovation within that space.[19]

TIPS TO INCREASE SKILL AS AN EXPERIMENTER

Perfectionist?
Balance thought with action.

CURE ANALYSIS PARALYSIS

Break out of your examine-it-to-death mode and just do it. If you find yourself holding back acting because you don't have all the information, it's likely that you want to improve your confidence to avoid criticism. Remember that anyone with 100% of the information will make good decisions, but when was the last time you had that luxury? The real test is who can act the soonest with a reasonable amount, but not all, of the data. Some studies suggest successful general managers are about 65% correct. Learn to make smaller decisions more quickly. This will make it easier for you to change course along the way to the correct decision.

CALM YOUR INNER WORRIER

You may get stuck in analysis mode because you are a chronic worrier who focuses on the downsides of action. Write down your worries, and for each one, write down the upside (a pro for each con). Once you consider both sides of the issue, you should be more willing to take action. Virtually any conceivable action has a downside, but it has an upside as well. Act, get feedback on the results, refine, and act again.

TURN THE MONUMENTAL INTO THE MANAGEABLE

Experimenting with a new idea, process, or any change involves pushing the envelope and taking chances. Doing those things inevitably leads to more misfires and mistakes. Research says that successful executives have made more mistakes in their careers than those who didn't make it. Start small so you can recover more quickly. Go for small wins. Create a rough prototype to visualize your idea. Remember, it shouldn't even be close to perfect, just formed enough so it provides a baseline to build from. Don't blast into a major task to prove your boldness. Break it down into smaller tasks. Take the easiest one for you first. Then build up to the tougher ones. Review each one to see

20

what you did well and not well, and set goals so you'll do something differently and better each time. End up accomplishing the big goal and taking the bold action. Challenge yourself. See how creative you can be in taking action a number of different ways.

 Don't mistake recklessness for proactivity when it comes to experimenting. In order to ensure the smoothest start and get as much buy-in as possible to your ideas up front, be sure to balance forging ahead with proper analysis and problem-solving due process.

RESOURCES TO LEARN MORE

Bregman, P. (2012, February 9). How to start the big project you've been putting off. *Harvard Business Review.*

Pychyl, T. A. (2008, March 26). Just get started. *Psychology Today.*

Afraid to fail?
Keep it in perspective.

ACCEPT THAT MOST INNOVATIONS FAIL

The most successful innovators found their eventual success through sheer quantity of tries and learning from failure. Studies show that 80% of innovations occur in the wrong place, are created by the wrong people (dye makers developed detergent, Post-it® Notes was a failed glue experiment, Teflon® was created by mistake), and 30%–50% of technical innovations fail in tests within the company. Even among those that make it to the marketplace, 70%–90% fail. The bottom line on change is a 95% failure rate, and the most successful innovators try lots of quick, inexpensive experiments to increase the chances of success. Try lots of quick, low-impact experiments to increase the chances of success. For example, try five ways to test a product rather than one big carefully planned one. Look for something common in the failure that is never present when there is a success. Let the plan evolve from the tests.

BE PHILOSOPHICAL ABOUT FAILURE/CRITICISM

After all, most innovations fail, most proposals fail, most change efforts fail, anything worth doing takes repeated effort. To increase learning from your mistakes, design feedback loops to be as immediate as possible. Involve others. The faster and the more frequent the cycles, the more opportunities to learn. There will be many mistakes and failures; after all, since you're not sure, it's very likely no one else knows what to do either. They just have a right to comment on your errors. The best tack when confronted with a mistake is to say, "What can we learn from this?"

20

 Treating failures and mistakes as chances to learn is a good strategy, but make sure it doesn't turn into a crutch. At some point, you need to draw a line in the sand and ask a different kind of hard question: "Is there more to be learned here or is it time to pack it in?"

DON'T GO IT ALONE

When you're in the throes of experimenting, you're bound to experience lots of setbacks. It helps to have a people support system. Brain research shows that what helps us be resilient in the face of disappointment is having a social network—not in the technology sense (though social networks are certainly helpful), but in the sense of staying connected to others. So make sure to engage others in the experimentation process. You can do this directly by delegating some of the experimenting tasks to others. Remember, the more people you have on board, the more tries you can make in a shorter amount of time. Indirectly, establish a go-to person whom you can commiserate with before, during, and after each try. By including others, you give yourself a safety net which will make you more at ease when those inevitable setbacks come your way.

RESOURCES TO LEARN MORE

Axelrod, A. (2008). *Edison on innovation: 102 Lessons in creativity for business and beyond.* San Francisco, CA: Jossey-Bass.

Kelley, T., & Littman, J. (2005). *The ten faces of innovation: Strategies for heightening creativity.* London, England: Profile Books Ltd.

Tend to avoid trying out the new?
Think and act differently.

TAP INTO YOUR PASSION

If you find yourself lacking motivation or commitment to be the lead on trying out new ideas, look around you and ask what's your passion? What do you have enthusiasm for or what truly needs to be done? Identify it. Appoint yourself as champion. Throw out trial balloons to other units/groups to see if your notion strikes a chord or solves a common problem. Find someone with an experimenter track record to go in with you. Bring in a heavy expert or someone with political clout to help you get traction. Plant seeds with others at every opportunity.

GET AWAY FROM YOUR FAVORITE SOLUTIONS

They interfere with growth and change. Decide what you would most likely do, then don't do it. Carve out some time—talk with others, look for parallels in other organizations, talk to an expert in an unrelated field, pick some unusual or odd facts about the problem you're facing and see what they signal, brainstorm with a one-time problem-solving group. Don't restrict your solution space. Creativity requires combining two things previously unconnected or changing how we look at them. It also requires generating

20

ideas without judging them initially. People who do this well are atypical as well—they may be playful, contrary, and averse to many rules. You may have to buffer them somewhat and give them some room. You won't get anything new by following the normal set-a-goal-and-time-schedule approach.

SHOW SOME PATIENCE
The flip side of analysis paralysis is rushing to get to the outcome and not having patience for the hard slogging that comes with trying, failing, course correcting, and trying again. The style that chills experimenting the most is the results-driven, time-short, and impatient person. If you focus too much on short-term results, it also means you'll have more of a tendency to take the first close-enough solution that comes along. Or look to abandon new ideas before they've had a chance to really be tried. Impatient people don't wait that long. Slow down. Discipline yourself to pause for enough time to let the idea get vetted through trial and error before calling it a lost cause.

RESOURCES TO LEARN MORE
Girard, L. (2012). Five creativity exercises to find your passion. *Entrepreneur.*
Kelley, T., & Littman, J. (2005). *The ten faces of innovation: Strategies for heightening creativity.* London, England: Profile Books Ltd.

ASSIGNMENTS TO PRACTICE SKILL
Insert yourself into a situation where you can help manage a crisis or change. This will require trying lots of new things fast to get to a viable resolution.

Relaunch an existing product or service that's not doing well by trying things not tried before. Or take on a tough and undoable project, one where others who have tried it have failed. In this environment, you're likely to have support for experimenting with unvetted ideas since it's obvious the "usual suspect" solutions haven't worked.

Work on a team that has to integrate diverse systems (move from using five computer platforms into one), processes (integrating a distinct, stand-alone quality assurance process into a product development process, for instance), or procedures (five disparate, escalated customer complaint procedures into one) across decentralized and/or dispersed units where you have to find the most common solution. You'll have to experiment with different combinations and prototypes to come up with the best solution for all.

20

TAKE TIME TO REFLECT...

Here are some questions to reflect on as you focus on being an Experimenter. Think about how you might answer these today and how, through using the tips in this chapter, you might achieve a better result in the future.

How well do you exploit your mistakes as opportunities to learn and improve? What do you do after the discovery of a mistake to capture what you learned? How do you ensure that you leverage this learning in the future? What will you start doing to better capitalize on your errors?

Do you find yourself able to generate lots of new ideas but hit a mental roadblock when the question turns to how to put it into practice? What would you gain by taking just one of those and testing it out, maybe in private or with small stakes? How would that self-pilot build your confidence to try bigger things?

What did you learn as a result of going through an experience that you could not have achieved in any other way? How would you communicate this learning to others? What was it about the experience that was so important?

A life spent making mistakes is not only more honorable, but more useful than a life spent doing nothing.

George Bernard Shaw
Irish essayist, playwright, and literary critic

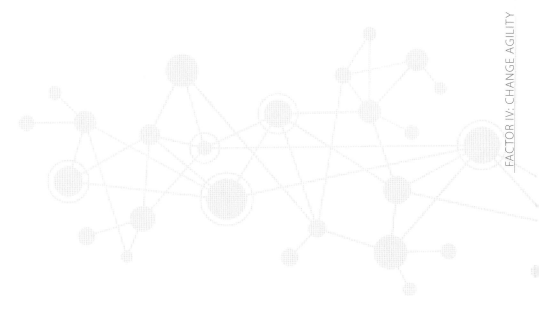

20

Innovation
Manager

Creative ideas, no matter how promising, won't amount to much unless they can be transformed into something tangible. The ability to think through and manage innovation is different from ordinary planning and execution. It's also harder to find. Research shows that managing innovation is a rare skill but one that organizations are seeking more and more. Being an Innovation Manager starts with knowing what sells and why. What more do your customers want? What do your non-customers want that they don't find in your offerings? Then you need to be able to sift through creative ideas and find the golden nugget—the idea that has the highest likelihood of success. Innovation Managers are able to take the raw idea and manage its transition into a successful something (product, service) in the marketplace. To do this well, you need to understand the creative process and the high failure rates associated with innovation. To know how to maneuver through the organizational maze so your execution efforts aren't sabotaged. Being able to find and then implement the new, different, and unique is what fuels innovation.

Great ideas need landing gear as well as wings.

General C. D. Jackson
American Special Assistant to President Eisenhower and publisher of *Fortune* magazine

21

SKILLED

Is able to take a creative idea and put it into practice

Can navigate through formal and informal channels to implement new ideas

Is both team and organizationally savvy

Will try more than one approach to bring a creative idea to life

Can project the steps needed to execute on innovations

Is not deterred by failures in implementing the new

LESS SKILLED

Has difficulty implementing ideas

May have trouble with the process of innovation

Doesn't understand how organizations work

Has difficulty securing and mobilizing resources

Doesn't anticipate the problems that will arise

Doesn't follow an orderly method of setting goals and laying out work

OVERUSE OF SKILL

May get too far out in front of others in thinking and planning

May push through innovations without consideration of people's concerns

Has a bias for implementing new ideas; undervalues established processes

SOME POSSIBLE CAUSES OF LOWER SKILL

Causes help explain "why" a person may have trouble in this dimension. When seeking to increase skill, it's helpful to consider how these might play out in certain situations. And remember that all of these can be addressed if you are motivated to do so.

Avoids conflict

Dislikes risk

Doesn't like to be out front leading

Impatient

Too comfortable with what is

Not inspiring

Not politically savvy

Not resourceful

Not well networked

Not well organized

DEVELOPMENTAL DIFFICULTY

When compared with other dimensions of Learning Agility, this dimension is **_harder_** to develop.

21

⭐ Does It Best

Steve Jobs is held up as a role model for many things, but an area where he really brought a unique skill set was as an Innovation Manager. Jobs wasn't the inventor at Apple—that was Steve Wozniak. Jobs didn't invent the digital audio player—a British engineer named Kane Kramer did. The smart phone was first conceptualized at IBM, not at Apple.[20] And the list goes on. The rare skill Jobs had was the ability to perfect other people's inventions—by understanding customers and what it takes to make innovations come to life in the marketplace.

TIPS TO INCREASE SKILL AS AN INNOVATION MANAGER

Trouble spotting the breakthrough idea from an array of good ideas? Pick the right innovation to manage.

UNDERSTAND YOUR MARKETS

Understand your markets historically, today, and, most importantly, tomorrow. Which new products succeeded and which failed? What do they buy today? Among your current customers, what more do they want and what are they willing to pay for? For those who did not buy your product or service, what was missing? What do your competitors have that you don't? What are the known future trends that will affect you? Aging of the population? Eating out? Electric cars? Green movement? Cyber security? What are some of the wilder possibilities? Fusion? Space travel? Subscribe to the *Futurist* magazine, a journal of the World Future Society. Talk to the strategic planners in your organization for their long-term forecasts. Consult your team. Talk to your key customers. What do they think their needs will be?

BECOME A STUDENT OF INNOVATION OUTSIDE YOUR FIELD

Don't limit your study of innovation just to the context of your own organization. Think of yourself as a customer. Look for and study new products you buy and use. Find out the process that was used to create it. Watch the History Channel's *Modern Marvels*. Listen to podcasts from Radiolab. Read Pulitzer Prize winning *The Soul of a New Machine* by Tracy Kidder to see how innovation happens from the inside. See how innovators use the past to predict the future. How several unrelated inventions came together to form a bigger one. Write down five things from your research that you can model in your own behavior, then put them into practice.

USE QUESTIONS TO PRIME THE IDEA PUMP

Solutions typically outweigh questions eight to one in problem-solving meetings. When it comes to innovation, this ratio is especially limiting. When brainstorming ideas, have the group ask more questions and spend half its time really looking at a problem statement. Have the group take a product/service you are dissatisfied with and represent it visually—flowchart it or use a series of pictures. Cut it up into its component pieces and reorder them. Ask how you could combine three pieces into one. Look for patterns. Pull fresh thinking into the group (use customers, people who know nothing about the area). Many studies have shown that the more diverse the group, the fresher the thinking. Innovation starts with lots of ideas and thorough examination of the problem.

RESOURCES TO LEARN MORE

Basulto, D. (2010, April 25). Before you innovate, understand the business model of your industry. Future Lab.

McKinney, P. (2012, February 17). Beyond the obvious: Killer questions that spark game-changing innovation [Video file].

Think managing innovation is a go-it-alone proposition? Get buy-in to fuel innovation efforts.

MAKE A COMPELLING CASE

Innovation is often like an orphan in an organization. Early in the process, resources will probably be tight. You will have to deal with other units and detractors. People will shy away from leaving their comfort zones. Studies show that establishing a sense of urgency early and getting it baked into the mind-set of the organization is critical. Be prepared to state the value again and again. What problem will it solve? How can it help the organization or other units? Think carefully about whom to go to and how to gain support. Appeal to the common good, trade something, and work to minimize negative effects on others. Work from the outside in. Determine the demands and interests of groups and individuals and appeal to those.

It's likely that you have a finite stack of chips to play to secure buy-in and resources for managing an innovation. So be mindful not to chase every idea like it's a bright, shiny object. Discriminate.

BE AN INFLUENCER

To move an innovation through the organization and ultimately into the marketplace, you are going to need people resources and other resources that you'll need to get through people. That means establishing and nurturing relationships. Relationships that work are built on equity and considering the impact on others. Things like influencing skills, understanding, and trading are the currencies to use. Don't just ask for things; find some common ground

21

where you can provide help, not just ask for it. What does the unit you're contacting need in the way of problem solving or information? Do you really know how they see the issue? Is it even important to them? How does what you're working on affect them? If it affects them negatively and they are balky, can you trade something, appeal to the common good, figure out some way to minimize the work or other impact (volunteering staff help, for example)?

INSPIRE TO INNOVATE

Innovation is tougher than work-as-usual. Support for the innovation will fade without regular injections of inspiration. The higher the level of ambiguity, the more our brain's anxiety center is put on high alert. So communicate often. Celebrate wins, measure progress in small steps, have members of the groups present promising results, establish common cause, reinforce often why this is important, set small checkpoints and little goals, and treat failures as exciting chances to learn how to do it better. If you hit roadblocks and sense support is waning, innovation experts recommend reestablishing a sense of urgency so the team stays grounded in the "why"—the payoff for their efforts.

 You may be crystal clear on the value of the innovation, but don't underestimate others' need for continued reinforcement. You may have to slow down at some points to go fast again. Stay attuned.

RESOURCES TO LEARN MORE

Adair, J. (2009). *Leadership for innovation: How to organize team creativity and harvest ideas.* Philadelphia, PA: Kogan Page Limited.

Hess, E. D. (2012, June 20). Creating an innovation culture: Accepting failure is necessary. *Forbes.*

No traction for good ideas?
Make ideas come to life in the organization and the marketplace.

LEARN HOW TO MOVE IDEAS THROUGH THE ORGANIZATION

Once an idea has been selected, you need to manage it through to the marketplace. Designing processes to get the job done most efficiently and effectively is a known science. Look to the principles of Total Quality Management, ISO, Six Sigma, and LEAN. Read up on each. Go to a workshop. Ask for help from the organizational effectiveness group in your organization or hire a consultant. Have the innovation team work with you to design the best way to proceed. Teams work better when they have a say in how things will be done.

WORK THE MAZE

To make that happen, you'll likely have to deal with many units outside your immediate area. Organizations can be complex mazes with many turns, dead ends, quick routes, and choices. In most organizations, the best path to get somewhere is almost never a straight line. Since organizations are made up of people, they become all that more complex. There are gatekeepers, expediters, blockers, resisters, guides, Good Samaritans, and influencers. Leading the way through the maze will be key to making your innovation a reality.

SPEED UP THE LEARNINGS CYCLE

The most successful innovators do it by sheer quantity and learning from failure. Don't expect to get it right the first time. This leads to safe and stale solutions. If you have trouble going back the second or third time to get something done, then switch approaches. Sometimes people get stuck in a repeating groove that's not working. Do something different next time. Think about multiple ways to get the same outcome. To increase learning, shorten the action phases of the innovation management process and insert feedback loops—aiming to make them as immediate as possible after any action. The more frequent the cycles, the more opportunities to learn.

> **RESOURCES TO LEARN MORE**
>
> Bossidy, L., & Charan, R. (with Burck, C.). (2002). *Execution: The discipline of getting things done.* New York, NY: Crown Business.
>
> Govindarajan, V., & Trimble, C. (2010). *The other side of innovation: Solving the execution challenge.* Boston, MA: Harvard Business School Press.

ASSIGNMENTS TO PRACTICE SKILL

Lead or become a key team member on a start-up effort which will require forging a new team and trying things for the first time on a tight timetable. The size of the start-up doesn't matter—it could be an athletic program, a suggestion system at work, or organizing a fundraiser, to name a few examples.

Lead a strategic, groundbreaking project for your organization where you will have to integrate the new into existing processes to bring the project to life.

Identify an unmet need and experiment with solutions that would fill the gap. You will need to discriminate between lots of good ideas on how to execute, get buy-in, and marshal resources.

21

TAKE TIME TO REFLECT...

Here are some questions to reflect on as you focus on being an Innovation Manager. Think about how you might answer these today and how, through using the tips in this chapter, you might achieve a better result in the future.

Have you ever had your efforts to implement a new idea squashed? How did that make you feel? Did it dissuade you from trying again? What could you have done differently that would have brought about a different outcome for your idea?

What do you do when you hit a roadblock when working on a project that involves people doing things differently? Who is usually in your corner to support you? Is it a small group? How do you make that group bigger and influential enough so roadblocks disappear?

When have you seen others limit their thinking to what is known and familiar? How has this affected their creativity and innovation? What did you do in this situation? What could you have done to remove the imaginary constraints?

....

Innovation distinguishes between a leader and a follower.

Steve Jobs
American entrepreneur and cofounder of Apple Inc. and Pixar Animation Studios

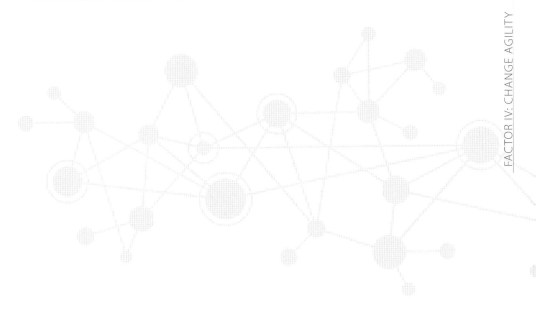

21

Comfort
Leading Change

Most significant innovations or change initiatives represent a deviation from the past. They represent a rallying call for a departure from business as usual. They require that people are going to have to think, talk, and act differently. Carrying the change banner can make you unpopular with some in the short-term and others in the long-term. Change is scary, frustrating, and worrisome for many. We like things to stay the same. After all, we're mostly wired to like the comfort zone and to nest build. And those who try to shake us out of our nests will feel our wrath. One reaction is to attack the change leader directly or, more likely, indirectly. Remove the change leader and the change goes away. Sabotage is common. To be a change champion, you have to be ready to pull some arrows from various places, including your back. Comfort Leading Change means you've learned to absorb this discomfort, honor the need of others to vent or resist, and still forge ahead with the change you know to be right.

Courage is resistance to fear, mastery of fear, not absence of fear.

Mark Twain
American humorist, satirist, lecturer, and writer

22

SKILLED

Philosophical about personal attacks

Knows that change is unsettling

Can take a lot of heat, even when it gets personal

Uses a balance of objectivity and empathy in dealing with the impact of change on others

Is not swayed by others' resistance to change

Willingly takes accountability for being the champion of a change

LESS SKILLED

May fold up under pressure or in the face of being in trouble with people

Wants to be liked by everyone

Ensures complete consensus before initiating change

May try too hard to please everyone

Unwilling to take the lead on unpopular stands

May be defensive and sensitive to criticism

OVERUSE OF SKILL

Marginalizes people's legitimate concerns about change

May come across as patronizing

Has a change-at-all-costs mentality

May be seen as cold and uncaring

SOME POSSIBLE CAUSES OF LOWER SKILL

Causes help explain "why" a person may have trouble in this dimension. When seeking to increase skill, it's helpful to consider how these might play out in certain situations. And remember that all of these can be addressed if you are motivated to do so.

Avoids conflict

Avoids criticism

Cares a lot about what people think

Defensive

Doesn't like to be first

Doesn't listen

Gets easily upset

Impatient with others

Not well networked

Prefers to share responsibility

Takes criticism personally

DEVELOPMENTAL DIFFICULTY

When compared with other dimensions of Learning Agility, this dimension is **harder** to develop.

22

⭐ Does It Best

In 1994, newly-appointed New York City police commissioner, William Bratton, inherited an unwieldy police force and a crime rate that was going nowhere but up. Yet in less than two years, Bratton significantly reversed the crime rate and established a productive operating model that is still largely in place today. His methods are now widely applied in other cities. How did he do it? He faced hurdle after hurdle and a lot of initial resistance from within the ranks of a skeptical, seen-it-all-before workforce. By making his officers experience for themselves what needed to change (subway-rider safety) and getting detractors on his side (appointing a veteran insider as his number two), Bratton was able to "take the heat" of resistance in order to make real and permanent change in the NYPD.[21]

TIPS TO INCREASE SKILL IN COMFORT LEADING CHANGE

Bracing for resistance?
Own the change from start to finish.

PREPARE IN ADVANCE
Leading is risky. Leading change is riskier. Championing change demands confidence in what you're saying, along with the humility that you might be wrong—one of life's paradoxes. While there are a lot of personal rewards for being out front on change, it puts you into the limelight. Look at what happens to political leaders and the scrutiny they face. People who choose to lead change have to be internally secure. Do you feel good about yourself? Can you defend to a critical audience the wisdom of what you're doing? To prepare to take the lead on a tough issue, work on your stand through mental interrogation until you can clearly state in a few sentences what your stand is and why you hold it. Build the business case. Prepare your case from the viewpoint of the problem it will solve for others. How do they win when the change is successful?

No matter how sound the reasoning behind the change or innovation you are leading is, change overload is a real phenomenon that can derail your best efforts. Be sure to properly gauge the appetite for change in the affected population and adjust accordingly.

ACKNOWLEDGE THE CHALLENGES OF CHANGE AND INNOVATION
Be up front about the difficulties that invariably accompany change of any significance. Don't hedge. Expect trouble and admit that 20%–40% of time will be spent debugging, fixing mistakes, and figuring out what went wrong. Be clear that you will treat each one as a chance to learn—document difficulties and learn from them. Without sounding like you're hedging, present it as a

work-in-progress to be improved over time. People will always say it should have been done differently. Even great leaders are wrong sometimes. They accept personal responsibility for errors and move on to lead some more. Don't let criticism prevent you from taking a stand. And don't let the possibility of being wrong hold you back from championing an innovation or change when you believe it's right.

MASTER THE RULES OF RESPONDING

When facing resisters to change, you'll likely face their questions. Lots of their questions. When that happens, keep it to any facts that are available. Think about the 10 most likely questions or criticisms you could face. "I don't think that will work." "Our customers won't go for it." Mentally rehearse how you might respond to questions. Some rules: Practice 10- to 30-second answers. Ask the questioner if that answered his/her question. Many spend too much time on the answers. Make sure you know what the question is. Many answer the wrong question. Ask one clarifying question if you're unsure: "Do you mean how would this product work in a foreign or domestic market?" You won't always win. But stay objective. Get it in your mind that questions are your friends because they reveal opportunities to solve problems and headline the difficulties you face. You just need five techniques to deal with them, including the dreaded but necessary "I don't know, but I'll find out and get back to you on that."

Being prepared is helpful, but appearing too rehearsed or having a set of pat answers is not. It can lead you to be perceived as not listening or, worse, patronizing. Show active listening, be nimble with your responses and, above all, stay authentic.

RESOURCES TO LEARN MORE

Harvard Business Review. (2011). *HBR's 10 must reads on change management* (including featured article "Leading Change," by John P. Kotter). Boston, MA: Harvard Business School Press.

Mortensen, K. (2008). *Persuasion IQ: The 10 skills you need to get exactly what you want.* New York, NY: AMACOM.

Looking to reduce the heat of leading change?
Build support for the change.

BE PREPARED FOR DETRACTORS AND RESISTERS

There will always be those who don't buy it, have seen it all before, haven't yet seen an innovation or change come to fruition. They may be private about it or come at you in public. Listen patiently to people's concerns, protect their feelings, but also reinforce the perspective of why the change is needed. Attack positions, not the people. Show patience toward the unconverted; keep things light by using humor constructively. To turn detractors into supporters, use the "keep your enemy closer" strategy. Bring a respected member of the

22

resistance cadre into the inner circle of your change team. Go for coffee once a week with your biggest critic. Rarely, you may have to pull a specific person aside and say, "I understand all your worries and have tried to respond to them, but the train is moving on. Are you on or off?"

 Don't get so enamored of your change that you become a bulldozer. You may get caught unawares by the ferocity of others' resistance, putting you and the change you champion at risk. Hear people out.

MANAGE THE MESSAGE

When leading and communicating change, you need to come across as confident and committed to the vision. But that doesn't mean bulldozing the people impacted. When confronted with resistance, look for common interests and underlying concerns. Almost all conflicts have common points that get lost in the heat of the battle. Try on their views for size—the emotion as well as the content. Ask yourself if you understand their feelings. Ask what they would do if they were in your shoes. See if you can restate each other's position and advocate it for a minute to get inside each other's place. Share of yourself freely, relate personal experiences or stories about why the change or innovation is needed. Welcome ideas, good and bad. Remember that any negative response is a positive if you learn from it.

GIVE OTHERS CHOICES

When a proposed change affects us personally, we often experience a highly visceral reaction. Part of this is due to feeling a loss of control. During the change process, the more you can emphasize what is still in a person's control and, when applicable, how the change will help them, the less resistance you're likely to face. So be flexible. To sell your views, clearly articulate the sense of urgency and "what's in it for them" attributes, but don't specify everything about how to get there. Give others room to maneuver. Present the outcomes, targets, and goals without the how to's. Your job is the *what* and the *why*. *How* changes can be implemented should be as open as possible. Studies show that people work harder when they have a sense of choice over how they accomplish the new and different.

22

RESOURCES TO LEARN MORE

Russell, J. E. A. (2010, September 13). Career coach: A key element of successfully managing change. *The Washington Post.*

Treasurer, B. (2008). *Courage goes to work: How to build backbones, boost performance, and get results.* San Francisco, CA: Berrett-Koehler Publishers.

Feeling the weight of change on your shoulders?
Take care of you.

KEEP IT IN PERSPECTIVE

When leading a change and facing people obstacles, remember that what is thwarting you isn't really about you, it's about others' resistance to change. About their propensity to want to nest build, to avoid loss of control, to want what's familiar, restore order, and ultimately protect themselves. As one change expert put it, "They want to be comfortable again, and you're in the way." Don't get in the fray, stay above it. As you go about the business of leading the change or innovation through to execution, act but reflect at the same time. "Who is defending the old way of doing things?" "What topics are triggering the most questions or challenges?" This will help you retain a dose of objectivity about what's going on with your initiative, how it's being adopted, and what's being directed at you.

HAVE A SAFE HARBOR OF YOUR OWN

When we're stressed, our brain's anxiety center kicks into high gear. If that happens, our decision-making ability and our ability to remain calm and measured are compromised. Establish a safe place (a friend's office, a park) or routine (a trip to the local coffee house, a daily walk) where you can go after a particularly harsh exchange or blow to your efforts. Find a trusted person (not from the change or innovation team) who can act as a support for you. The same research on what works best for conflict management—focus on the issue, not the person—also applies to your role as change leader or champion. It'll be healthier for you personally and professionally if you keep your identity separate from the change you are leading. Lead the change without becoming the face of, or synonymous with, the change.

STAY CALM IF THINGS GET HEATED

Sometimes your emotional reactions lead others to think you have problems with taking tough positions and stands. Worse, it gives them fodder to undercut your change efforts. When things get heated, what emotional reactions do you have? Do you show nervousness or non-verbals like increasing or wavering voice volume or fidgeting? Learn to recognize those as soon as they start. Ask a question to buy time. Pause. Or ask the person to tell you more about his/her point of view. Restate their position so they know you've heard them. You don't have to do anything to appease, just listen and accept that they are

22

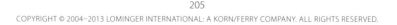

irritated. Often, their main objective is just to be heard. Your goal is to calm the situation so you can get back to a more reasonable discussion.

RESOURCES TO LEARN MORE

Adams, S. (2012, June 18). Eight ways goofing off can make you more productive. *Forbes*.

Warrell, M. (2008). *Find your courage: 12 Acts for becoming fearless at work and in life*. New York, NY: McGraw-Hill.

ASSIGNMENTS TO PRACTICE SKILL

Manage a crisis or high-profile, high-risk project that requires tough-minded decisions under tight time pressure with a low level of consultation and high visibility.

Manage a group of balky and resisting people through an unpopular change or project. You will need to be able to balance the noise of their concerns and be empathetic but still move forward with the project.

Handle a tough negotiation with an internal or external client or customer, or manage a dissatisfied internal or external customer; troubleshoot a performance or quality problem with a product or service.

TAKE TIME TO REFLECT...

Here are some questions to reflect on as you focus on Comfort Leading Change. Think about how you might answer these today and how, through using the tips in this chapter, you might achieve a better result in the future.

How do you motivate your team toward change? Where do you lean in terms of motivating versus pressuring? How might you use one approach (or a combination of both) more effectively?

Where are you currently fighting change? What is the reason for the resistance? What are you afraid of? What will it take for you to change your attitude and approach toward the change? How might this help you to deal effectively with others' resistance?

When have you been caught by surprise at the amount of resistance to change? What did you learn about the process, its impact, and the people involved? How did this help your understanding?

Where have you seen someone exhibit resistance or reluctance? What can you learn from their experience? What will you do to ensure you remain more open-minded?

There are two ways of meeting difficulties:
You alter the difficulties or you alter yourself to meet them.

Phyllis Bottome
British novelist

22

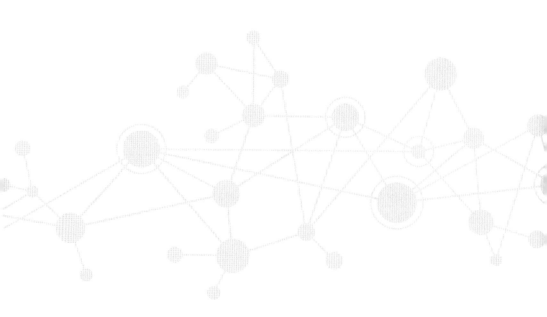

Results Agility

At first glance, Results Agility seems to be comprised of a relatively straightforward set of behaviors. Work hard. Make adjustments. Get results. End of story. Right? Look a bit closer and the nuances and interconnections reveal something more rich and complex. First, there are two critical subplots—getting results mostly on your own and getting results through others. For the results-through-self component, Results Agility starts with drive. Individuals high in Results Agility have a strong desire to achieve goals. They know that in order to accomplish extraordinary things, they need the will to push themselves hard. What distinguishes the high results agile person from ordinary performers is what happens when they face obstacles and unforeseen circumstances on the path to achieving their goals. That's where resourcefulness comes into play. And since most everything of significant and lasting value that's accomplished at work today involves others, the results agile person builds the best team to get a tough job done successfully. The results agile person uses presence to set the tone—exuding an aura of confidence and poise that stirs the belief in others that the impossible can be achieved. Presence, coupled with the ability to inspire others, enables belief to translate into action. When the passion and energy of a group converge around a common cause, amazing things can indeed happen. It all culminates in a proven ability to deliver against the odds. Of course, for the truly results agile person, there is no real sense of achieving success. Once they've reached the top of one peak, they are already plotting the course up the next mountain.

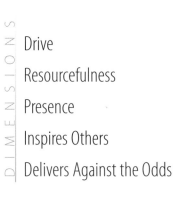

DIMENSIONS

Drive

Resourcefulness

Presence

Inspires Others

Delivers Against the Odds

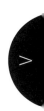

Drive

Many phrases attempt to capture what it means to demonstrate Drive. "Go for it." "Never surrender." "Reach for the stars." Whatever phrase resonates with you, one theme is consistent—that something powerful and intense is at work. Something capable of creating a big impact. Something that comes deep from within. Individuals high in Drive tap into this energy inside and channel it directly toward the outcomes they seek. Nurtured and sustained correctly, it provides sustainable fuel to overcome challenges and achieve at the highest levels. And the need for Drive has never been stronger. In fact, Drive is no longer a differentiator in the current fast-paced, ultra-competitive business environment. Both the rising demand and the ample supply have transformed it into a must-have skill. Simply put, you need to find your Drive and apply it to the utmost. Because challenges will not cease, sacrifices will continue to be demanded, and change will be constant. Imagine surviving, let alone thriving, without Drive.

In all human affairs there are efforts, and there are results, and the strength of the effort is the measure of the result.

James Allen
British writer and poet

23

SKILLED
Pushes self hard to accomplish goals and objectives
Strives for the highest levels of achievement
Is motivated by challenges
Continually stretches self to perform at a higher level
Thrives on multitasking

LESS SKILLED

Is content with meeting minimum goal requirements

Maintains a more easily manageable workload

Prefers familiar situations that favor his/her skill set

Has difficulty sustaining effort in the face of challenges

Prefers to work on one thing at a time

OVERUSE OF SKILL

Pushes self to the point of burnout

Pursues goals at a significant cost to self and/or others

Is unyielding in his/her efforts

Carries too much responsibility

Expects too much from self

SOME POSSIBLE CAUSES OF LOWER SKILL

Causes help explain "why" a person may have trouble in this dimension. When seeking to increase skill, it's helpful to consider how these might play out in certain situations. And remember that all of these can be addressed if you are motivated to do so.

Low need for achievement	Easily overwhelmed
Not goal oriented	Narrow comfort zone
Lacks ambition	Undisciplined
Relaxed standards	Disengaged
Low self-confidence	Feels entitled
Tires easily	Difficulty balancing priorities

DEVELOPMENTAL DIFFICULTY

When compared with other dimensions of Learning Agility, this dimension is **_easier_** to develop.

23

Did You Know?

Drive is by far the highest-rated dimension of Learning Agility in terms of skill. It is highly valued and most people excel at it. If Drive is among your less skilled dimensions of Learning Agility, then you should be aware of how conspicuous its absence may be and how it might affect others' perceptions of you. The good news is, it is also among the easiest Learning Agility dimensions to develop. Drive comes from within, and the solution to strengthening it begins and ends with you. Better to start now. Sooner than later, you will feel the demand to demonstrate a high level of drive. If yours is not sustainable, or there's little there to begin with, it will be hard to keep up with the challenges you face.

TIPS TO INCREASE SKILL IN DRIVE

Feeling lackluster?
Give yourself a motivation makeover.

FOCUS ON YOUR INTERESTS
Uncover what motivates you and then fuel your drive from within. Make a list of what you like to do and don't like to do. Do your least preferred activities first. Focus not on the activity but on your sense of accomplishment. Then concentrate on doing at least a few things you like each day. Take note of what others are doing. See if you can delegate or trade for more desirable activities. If what you like to do isn't already part of your job, volunteer for task forces and projects that would be more interesting for you.

REVISIT YOUR PRIORITIES
Shift your energy to what really matters. Some people get results but don't focus on the most important priorities. Darting from task to task, working on whatever comes up, can be draining. Successful managers, by contrast, typically spend half their time on two or three key priorities. They give attention, but not too much, to lesser priorities. The key questions are: What should you be spending half your time on? Can you name five priorities that are less critical than these? If you can't, then you are not differentiating well.

LEARN THE FACTS ABOUT SUCCESS
If you feel like your efforts aren't getting you anywhere, perhaps you don't know how successful careers are really built. What has staying power is performing in a variety of jobs (not more of the same jobs), having a few notable strengths, and seeking new tasks that you don't know how to do. A successful career is built on stress and newness. Not slogging your way through the same old problems. Talk to some successful people in your organization and hear how

23

random their careers likely have been. Read *The Lessons of Experience, High Flyers,* and *Breaking the Glass Ceiling* to see how successful executives grew over time.

RESOURCES TO LEARN MORE

Lowe, T., & Giuliani, R. (2009). *Get motivated! Overcome any obstacle, achieve any goal and accelerate your success with motivational DNA.* New York, NY: Doubleday Publishing.

Pink, D. (2009, August 25). The puzzle of motivation [Video file].

Playing it safe?
Challenge yourself.

DO DIFFERENT THINGS

Find an activity that goes against your natural interests and try it. Up your risk comfort. Start small so you can recover quickly. Pick a few smaller tasks or challenges and build the skill bit by bit. For example, if strategic thinking is a stretch skill for you, write a strategic plan for your unit and show it to people to get feedback. Then write a second draft. You can also stretch yourself outside work. Devise a strategy for turning one of your hobbies (i.e., photography) into a business.

TAKE ON A TOUGH ASSIGNMENT

Many people turn down career opportunities based upon current life comforts, only to regret it later when they are passed by. Perhaps you love what you do now and can't imagine doing anything else. The problem with that is needs change, and if you don't, your prospects are not bright. That scary and unappealing new job will add new skills and variety to your resume at the least. Most successful people have taken any number of jobs which didn't appeal but which did broaden them.

If you are at risk for burnout, periodically stop to check your vitals. Get control over your drive before it enters the danger zone. Asking yourself questions helps gain proper perspective. Why am I pushing myself so hard? What are the consequences? Does this match the pattern of other times where I've gone too far? How could I leverage others' drive?

TAKE MORE RISKS

Research indicates that more successful people have made more mistakes than the less successful. You can't learn anything if you're not trying anything new. Start small, experiment a bit. Go for small wins so you can recover quickly if you miss and, more importantly, learn from the results. Start with the easiest challenge, then work up to the tougher ones. Seek feedback and open yourself up to new learning along the way.

23

RESOURCES TO LEARN MORE

Geller, L. (2012, July 25). Getting out of your comfort zone. *Forbes*.

Masie, E. (2007, August 24). Three cheers for stretch assignments. *Chief Learning Officer*.

Frustrated easily?
Master the essentials of maintaining Drive.

CREATE POWERFUL GOALS

Use goals for yourself and others to build passion and drive. Almost everyone is motivated by achieving goals. Especially if they have had a hand in setting them. Make goals small and reasonably achievable. Set incremental goals or process goals. Don't just set the outcome or end goals. Create a goal process so there can be a lot of celebrating along the way. The scientific principles of goal setting are well established. Take a course on goal setting. No time? Read the key works of Edwin Locke and Gary Latham.

DON'T TRY TO GET IT RIGHT THE FIRST TIME

If a situation is ambiguous, be incremental. Make some small decisions and get instant feedback. Expect things to go wrong. Don't get frustrated when they do. Treat mistakes and failures as ways to learn. Focus on your third or fourth try, not the first. If you keep coming up short on results, take solace in the wisdom of Thomas Edison—you haven't failed, you've just discovered the various ways that don't work.

VARY YOUR APPROACH

Are you prone to give up on tough or repetitive tasks? Have trouble going back the second and third time? Lose motivation when you hit obstacles? Trouble making that last push to get it over the top? Changing things up, even just a little, can spark new energy. Commit yourself to switching approaches. Regardless of the outcome of your efforts, do something totally different next time. Strive to find five different ways to get the same outcome. Be prepared to do them all when obstacles arise. Task trade with someone who has your problem. Work on each other's tasks. Developing versatility keeps you fresh and poised to tackle the unexpected.

RESOURCES TO LEARN MORE

Harvard Business School Press. (2009). *Setting goals* (Pocket Mentor). Boston, MA: Author.

Maxwell, J. C. (2003). *Thinking for a change: 11 Ways highly successful people approach life and work*. New York, NY: Warner Books, Inc.

23

ASSIGNMENTS TO PRACTICE SKILL

Take on an important challenge where others' previous efforts have fallen short of success. Summon the motivation and energy needed to begin the journey and press on through the challenges and setbacks you are likely to face.

Go large. Stretch your capacity for hard work and multitasking by taking on a bigger region, a bigger budget, or a higher number of locations.

Take on a responsibility that you dislike or even hate doing. The experience will build up your focus and resilience when it comes to tackling go-against-the-grain (GAG) assignments.

TAKE TIME TO REFLECT...

Here are some questions to reflect on as you focus on Drive. Think about how you might answer these today and how, through using the tips in this chapter, you might achieve a better result in the future.

How well articulated are your goals? Which of your goals do you need to spend more time on defining them? How clearly have you spelled out what success will look like, how you will measure it, and how you will reach it? Who will you need support from in order to achieve these goals?

What do you typically do when faced with a challenge? Do you view it as an opportunity to stretch your skills and learn? Do you prefer activities that reinforce your well-developed strengths? What will you do to get out of your comfort zone?

Where do you see a gap between what you know to be excellence and seeing excellence realized? How can you lessen these gaps? What action steps will you take to make this happen?

When has your hard work and sacrifice yielded the most favorable rewards? What kept you going? How can you leverage what you learned from that experience and apply it to new situations?

....

Energy and persistence conquer all things.

Benjamin Franklin
American scientist, author, inventor, statesman, and diplomat

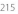
23

Resourcefulness

Resourcefulness is about finding a way. Not *the* way, but *a* way—in some cases, *any* way. With Resourcefulness, obstacles and setbacks are merely something to be navigated. Over, under, around, or through, the resourceful person finds a way. Resourceful individuals cultivate multiple ways of solving problems over time and can also devise new approaches at a moment's notice because they've learned from their past experiences. When a tough new situation comes their way, the resourceful person has a file bursting with different approaches to draw upon. Fluid in thought and action, they don't take a fixed view of situations and don't stubbornly apply one-size-fits-all solutions. The unexpected and insufficient inspires rather than frustrates. Your Resourcefulness is an indispensable asset in an increasingly VUCA (volatile, uncertain, complex, and ambiguous) world where things don't go as planned, you are forced to do more with less, and obstacles are omnipresent.

We will either find a way, or make one.

Hannibal
Carthaginian politician and military commander (247 BCE – 182 BCE)

24

SKILLED

Gets the most out of available resources

Adapts quickly to changing circumstances

Cleverly navigates obstacles and constraints

Knows where and who to go to for help

Tries new approaches when initial way isn't successful

LESS SKILLED

Gets frustrated when things don't go as planned

Sticks with one chosen approach

Relies on the same resources over and over

Complains about not having enough resources

Has difficulty figuring out where to get resources

OVERUSE OF SKILL

Stretches available resources beyond capacity

Implements stop-gap solutions that don't last

Diverts too quickly from planned approach

Deviates too far from accepted practices

Hoards resources from others

SOME POSSIBLE CAUSES OF LOWER SKILL

Causes help explain "why" a person may have trouble in this dimension. When seeking to increase skill, it's helpful to consider how these might play out in certain situations. And remember that all of these can be addressed if you are motivated to do so.

Rigid mind-set

Narrow perspective

Low creativity

Limited experience base

Low risk orientation

Defeatist attitude

Low threshold for frustration

Stubbornly upholds rules/traditions

Highly conscientious

Excessive loyalty

Hesitant to bargain/negotiate

DEVELOPMENTAL DIFFICULTY

When compared with other dimensions of Learning Agility, this dimension is **moderately difficult** to develop.

24

🔍 Did You Know?

Resourcefulness is such an integral part of life in bustling India, it has given rise to a particularly Indian form of innovation known as *jugaad*. Tracing its popular roots to Indian farmers' construction of jitney-like vehicles from scrap wood and irrigation pump motors, jugaad has found its way into the management lexicon as companies increasingly turn to "frugal innovation" practices to fuel their R&D operations. Recent innovations in everything from cars to medical devices to mobile banking all owe some inspiration to the principles of jugaad.

TIPS TO INCREASE SKILL IN RESOURCEFULNESS

Struggling to find a solution?
Learn real-time innovation.

KEEP LEARNING AS YOU GO

First time and tough situations call for resourcefulness. First time means you haven't done exactly this before. So, first, define what it is that needs to be done. Then set final and interim goals and measures. Next, try to lay out the work in incremental steps with the full expectation that this will change and evolve over time. Then find and bargain for the resources you will need to perform. Get the support you need and rally the team that will be working on the project. Delegate as much as possible. Celebrate incremental gains. Experiment and expect some false paths and mistakes. Have a process for instant correction of the plan. Make things up as you go. Expect the unexpected. All the while, relentlessly drive toward the original goals.

Improvising comes so naturally for some that it forms a dangerous habit. There eventually comes a time when your plan isn't quick enough, isn't clever enough to get you out of a jam. Spare yourself the potential disaster. Trust your versatility and adaptability but don't rely on it. Offset the risks with a judicious amount of foresight and planning.

TRY DIFFERENT SOLUTIONS AND LEARN FROM THE RESULTS

Don't expect to get it right the first time. A low-risk, perfectionist mind-set leads to safe and stale solutions. Many studies show that the second or third try is when we really understand the underlying dynamics of problems. To increase learning, shorten your action time and get feedback loops—aiming to make them as immediate as possible. The more frequent the cycles, the more opportunities to learn; if we do something in each of three days instead of one thing every three days, we triple our learning opportunities and increase our chances of finding the right answer.

24

DO QUICK EXPERIMENTS AND TRIALS

Studies show that 80% of innovations occur in the wrong place, are created by the wrong people (dye makers developed detergent; Post-it® Notes was an error in a glue formula) and 30%–50% of technical innovations fail in tests within the company. Even among those that make it to the marketplace, 70%–90% fail. The bottom line on change is a 95% failure rate. The most successful innovators try lots of quick, inexpensive experiments. Rapid and continual experimenting increases your chances of quickly achieving the 5% success rate.

RESOURCES TO LEARN MORE

Baldoni, J. (2010, January 13). The importance of resourcefulness. *Harvard Business Review.*

Laufenberg, D. (2010, December). How to learn? From mistakes [Video file].

Difficulty accessing resources?
Master the organizational maze.

STUDY HOW ORGANIZATIONS WORK

Organizations can be complex mazes with many turns, dead ends, quick routes, and seemingly endless choices. In most organizations, the best path to get somewhere is almost never a straight line. There is a formal organization— the one on the organization chart—where the path may look straight, and then there is the informal organization, where all paths are zigzagged. Since organizations are staffed with people, they become all that more complex. There are gatekeepers, expediters, stoppers, resisters, guides, Good Samaritans, and influencers. All of these types live in the maze. The key to successful maneuvering through complex organizations is to find your way through the maze in the least amount of time making the least noise. The best way to do that is to accept the complexity of organizations rather than fighting it, and learn to be a maze-bright person. *Patience is also important.* Maneuvering through the maze includes stopping once in a while to let things run their course.

LEARN TO READ THE POLITICAL LANDSCAPE

Organizations, no matter the type, are full of politics. They are populated with strong egos and empire-driven individuals. Some political agendas are plain to see while others are cleverly disguised. In this complex and confusing environment, it is easy to step into political traps and dead ends. Being politically savvy requires knowing the organization. This includes both knowing how to get things done and knowing who to rely on for expediting things. Identify who the major gatekeepers are who control the flow of resources, information, and decisions. Get to know them and nurture strong,

24

lasting relationships. Also identify who the major resisters and stoppers are, and try to avoid or sidestep them.

RALLY SUPPORT

Share your goals with the people you need to support you. Try to get their input. People who are asked for input tend to cooperate more than people who are not asked. Figure out how the people who support your goals can win along with you. It's easier to get things done when everybody is pulling in the same direction. It's easier to perform when you have all the tools and resources you need. It's easier to get things done when everyone you need in your corner is supportive and pulling for you.

RESOURCES TO LEARN MORE

Birkinshaw, J. (2012). *Reinventing management: Smarter choices for getting work done.* San Francisco, CA: Jossey-Bass.

Goldstein, M., & Read, P. (2009). *Games at work: How to recognize and reduce office politics.* San Francisco, CA: Jossey-Bass.

Trying to do it all yourself?
Leverage others' motivation and strengths.

BECOME A STUDENT OF THE PEOPLE AROUND YOU

First, try to outline their strengths and weakness, their preferences and beliefs. Watch out for traps—it is rarely general intelligence or pure personality that spells the difference in people. Most people are smart enough, and many personality characteristics don't matter that much for performance. Second, look below surface descriptions of smart, approachable, technically skilled people to get at specifics. Then try to predict ahead of time what they would do in specific circumstances. What percent of the time are your predictions correct? Try to increase the percent over time.

MATCH PEOPLE TO TASK REQUIREMENTS

People are different; tasks are different. People have different strengths and have different levels of knowledge and experience. Instead of thinking of everyone as equal, think of them as different. Equal treatment is really giving each person tasks to do that match their capacities. Look at the success profile of each assignment and line it up with the capabilities of each person. Assign things based upon that match.

KNOW AND PLAY THE MOTIVATION ODDS

According to research by Renwick and Lawler, the top motivators at work are (1) job challenge, (2) accomplishing something worthwhile, (3) learning new things, (4) personal development, and (5) autonomy. Pay (12th), friendliness (14th), praise (15th), or chance of promotion (17th) are not insignificant but are superficial compared with the more powerful motivators. Provide challenges, paint pictures of why this is worthwhile, create a common mind-set, set up chances to learn and grow, and provide autonomy, and you'll hit the vast majority of people's hot buttons.

RESOURCES TO LEARN MORE

Kruse, K. (2012). *Employee engagement 2.0: How to motivate your team for high performance (A real-world guide for busy managers)*. Richboro, PA: The Kruse Group.

Nauert, R. (2012, October 3). Work is rewarding when personal traits match job. *Psych Central*.

ASSIGNMENTS TO PRACTICE SKILL

Begin something new from scratch which will require you to form a new team and initiate a number of simultaneous actions under a tight time frame. You will likely need to practice resilience when facing the unexpected and possibly unpleasant that comes with any new venture.

Lead an underresourced project that requires you to adapt from the "normal" ways of doing things and may also require you to bargain and trade with others to get what you need to succeed.

Plan an off-site meeting, conference, convention, trade show, or event. You will almost certainly encounter obstacles and constraints and will need to quickly identify the right resources to help you.

24

TAKE TIME TO REFLECT...

Here are some questions to reflect on as you focus on Resourcefulness. Think about how you might answer these today and how, through using the tips in this chapter, you might achieve a better result in the future.

How do you react to situations that do not unfold smoothly? How do you deal with the "potholes" in the road of life? What would you like to do differently in how you approach or react to challenges?

What points of your career arose from need or desperation? How did innovation or resourcefulness manifest itself? What can you take from that situation to other aspects of work?

When have you experimented with a novel approach that resulted in success? What did it take for you to experiment versus doing what had always been done? How did you navigate this idea? What did you learn from the experience?

What have you postponed because you lacked the resources you thought you needed? What progress could you make with the resources that you have? How could you better leverage your existing resources to garner support for your cause? What is one step you can take today that will get you closer to your goal?

Adversity is just change that we haven't adapted ourselves to yet.

Aimee Mullins
American athlete, actress, fashion model, and Paralympian

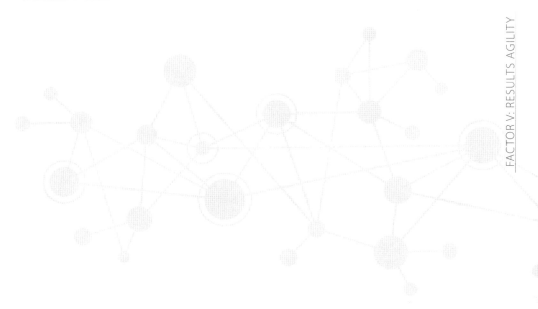

24

Presence

Presence is a particular form of personal brand. It's your way of saying to everyone, "You can count on me." Presence shows on the outside but it comes from the inside. When you feel equipped to face a new challenge because you've amassed learnings from past challenges, it's easier to demonstrate that to others. Presence takes shape in many forms. It can be brash and bold and it can be subtle and subdued. But for it to be effective, it has to be your own. While you might have to adapt or adopt certain behaviors to strengthen your Presence, there needs to be something authentic at the core. A false pretense doesn't inspire confidence, it only adds to the anxiety. A true and effective Presence sets the stage for making the impossible possible. It encourages others to look beyond constraints and pursue fresh possibilities. Your Presence is often forged in the toughest of circumstances, but endures through both good times and bad. Establish the Presence you want others to remember you by.

Keep your fears to yourself, but share your courage with others.

Robert Louis Stevenson
Scottish essayist, poet, and novelist

SKILLED

Maintains focus and composure in stressful circumstances

Projects confidence and poise

Faces challenges head-on

Steps to the forefront in a crisis

Puts others at ease

LESS SKILLED

Prefers to stay in the background

Is unnerved by challenging circumstances

Freezes in the face of uncertainty

Second-guesses self

Immediately looks to others for answers in a crisis

OVERUSE OF SKILL

Is overly self-confident

Creates a false sense of calm and security

Overshadows others

Is too concerned with his/her image

SOME POSSIBLE CAUSES OF LOWER SKILL

Causes help explain "why" a person may have trouble in this dimension. When seeking to increase skill, it's helpful to consider how these might play out in certain situations. And remember that all of these can be addressed if you are motivated to do so.

Shy

Low self-confidence

Fears failure/rejection

Low threshold for stress

Quick to follow; hesitant to lead

Low composure

Favors thinking over action

Difficulty with ambiguity

Difficulty connecting with others

Too understated

Low self-awareness

DEVELOPMENTAL DIFFICULTY

When compared with other dimensions of Learning Agility, this dimension is **_moderately difficult_** to develop.

⭐ Does It Best

Great presence doesn't mean you have to possess an athlete's build and a booming voice. Throughout history, there have been leaders renowned for their presence who were diminutive, even frail, in their appearance. Vaclav Havel. Mother Teresa. Picasso. Joan of Arc. Gandhi. New York's legendary mayor, Fiorello LaGuardia. By tapping into their values, creativity, and dreams, they established a charisma and an impact that far exceeded their stature.

TIPS TO INCREASE SKILL IN PRESENCE

Nerves getting the better of you?
Tame your insides.

PREPARE IN ADVANCE

Leading is risky. You have to defend what you're doing, so convince yourself first that you are on the right track. Be prepared to explain again and again. Prepare to attract criticism from detractors, from those unsettled by change, and from those who will always say it could have been done differently, better, and cheaper. To ready yourself for this, think about the 10 objections that will come up and mentally rehearse how you will reply. Listen patiently to people's concerns, acknowledge them, then explain why you think the change will be beneficial. Attack positions but not people. Role-play your approach with someone willing to test you and give you honest feedback.

BUILD UP YOUR CONFIDENCE

Take a course or work with a mentor or coach to build your confidence in one area at a time. In addition to building skill, focus on the strengths you do have. Think of ways you can use them to your benefit and cover for areas where you are weaker. If you're an expert in an area, imagine yourself calmly delivering key points to establish your confidence and put others at ease. If you are particularly concerned with your skills in a certain area, seek opportunities outside of work to practice and get feedback. Then gradually transfer your new learning to your job. Be patient. Research shows that it can take up to eight positive instances of a new behavior before people begin to alter their views and question the previous negative or unskilled behavior.

Is your display of confidence bordering on arrogance? Try moving in the opposite direction and show a little vulnerability. A small dose of weakness can actually strengthen your leadership connection to others.

RECHARGE YOURSELF

If you're stressed and worn out by what you're doing, find something to be enthusiastic about. Appoint yourself as champion of the change. Throw out trial balloons to see if your notion spurs some interest. Find an experimenter to go in with you. Bring in a heavy expert. Plant seeds at every opportunity. Then channel your restored energy and confidence into different problems and pursuits.

RESOURCES TO LEARN MORE

Andersen, E. (2012, July 23). 3 Simple ways to discover your passion. *Forbes*.

Goldsmith, B. (2010). *100 Ways to boost your self-confidence: Believe in yourself and others will too*. Franklins Lakes, NJ: The Career Press.

Projecting a low impact Presence?
Refashion your personal brand.

STUDY LEADERS WITH STRONG PRESENCE

Leading is greatly aided by presence. You have to look and sound like a leader. Study people who have a commanding presence. Who "own the room" when they're present. Pay attention to their voice modulation, change of pace, eye contact, gestures, and so on. Do you dress the part? Do you sound confident? Do you complain, or do you project an image of someone who solves problems? Giving presentations and looking the part is a well-known craft. Go to a course, join Toastmasters. Get coaching from an acting director. Act a scene in a pretend play called "Presence."

CHOOSE YOUR WORDS MORE CAREFULLY

Eliminate poor speech habits such as using the same words repeatedly, using filler words like "uh" and "you know," speaking too rapidly or forcefully, or going into so much detail that people can't follow what you're saying. Avoid condescending terms like "what you need to understand" or "this is the third time…." Both imply the receiver is either stupid or unwilling. Don't use words that are personal, blaming, or autocratic. Outline arguments. Know the three things you're trying to say and say them succinctly. Others can always ask questions if something is unclear.

25

STUDY WHAT GREAT ACTORS DO

Using acting as a model for building presence, there are several aspects of the stage performance that enter into the actor's skills:

- The first is the significance of the entrance. People tend to form short-term impressions based on little other than the manner of entrance, the physical characteristics of the actor, and the words and non-verbal behaviors in the first few moments. Think about the impression you want to leave. Visualize your entrance. Does it leave the message you intend. Do you look, act, and sound your intended presence?

- Next is establishing your voice. Voice has three elements. The first is the actual delivery voice. Volume. Tone. Speed. Language. Articulation. The second is non-verbals. Do your non-verbals (gestures, posture, facial expressions, movement) align with your message? The next is content. Are you confident and knowledgeable? Is it apparent that you know what you are talking about? Do you know your lines?

- The next element of presence is audience engagement. How do you intend to engage the audience? Is this going to be participative? Does the audience have a role? Do they know what it is you expect? Are you in command of your audience?

- The last element of presence is the exit. How do you intend to wrap things up? Do you have a strong close? Have you planned how you are going to end and finish by leaving your audience with the thoughts and conclusions you intended?

For the actor, these are the elements of creating a strong stage presence. Everything matters. Taken all together, they build presence. It's not that different in the world of work. One way or another, you're always on stage.

RESOURCES TO LEARN MORE

Koegel, T. J. (2007). *The exceptional presenter: A proven formula to open up and own the room.* Austin, TX: Greenleaf Book Group Press.

Stevenson, W. H., III. (2011, February). Cutting out filler words. Toastmasters.

Prone to gaffes and faux pas?
Understand your impact and seize the moment.

SEEK CRITICAL FEEDBACK

Others view people who seek critical feedback more positively. People who seek only positive feedback get the opposite response. The former shows willingness to improve. The latter is often seen as defensiveness and a disinterest in really knowing oneself. Disclose more. If you deny, minimize, or excuse away mistakes and shortcomings, take a chance and admit that you're imperfect like everyone else. Let your inside thoughts out in the open more often. Take personal responsibility. Admit mistakes matter-of-factly, inform everyone potentially affected, learn from it so the mistake isn't repeated, then move on. Research shows that successful people make lots of mistakes. All of this adds to a positive presence.

LISTEN MORE
Do you really know how others see the issue, or do you just tell and sell? Do you even know if it is important to them? Don't interrupt. Don't suggest words or solutions when they pause. Don't cut them off by saying, "I already know that," "I've heard that before," or the dreaded, "But I know that won't work." Be a two-way person. Practice reciprocity. Try to follow the rule of exchange. They get something, you get something. Build your presence by being more open, sharing, and giving.

FOCUS ON THE ESSENCE
When speaking to someone or a group, state your message or purpose in a single sentence, then outline your pitch around three to five things that support this thesis and that you want people to remember. Consider what someone should be able to say 15 minutes after you finish. Don't try to tell the audience all you know, even if they are well informed on the topic. You are giving a persuasive argument or communicating key information; it's not a lecture. Drowning people in detail will lose even the knowledgeable and the interested. Practice out loud. Writing out a pitch or argument isn't useful until you say it. Writing sounds stilted when spoken because the cadence of speech and sentence length is generally quite different.

RESOURCES TO LEARN MORE

Fenson, S. (2000, March 1). Want to be more effective? Learn to listen. *Inc.com*

London, M. (2003). *Job feedback: Giving, seeking, and using feedback for performance improvement*. Mahwah, NJ: Lawrence Erlbaum Associates, Inc.

ASSIGNMENTS TO PRACTICE SKILL

Seize the opportunity to lead others during a scary and unpredictable time. You will need to tap into the collective mood, but also establish the presence needed to center and stabilize others' feelings and perceptions.

Become a spokesperson to customers on a controversial issue. This will give you practice with carefully managing messages and demonstrating poise in handling the delicate balance of being sensitive to the needs of customers while simultaneously preserving the company's reputation.

Handle the fallout from an unpopular and/or unsuccessful initiative. This will require you to "take some heat" while also establishing confidence, and hope that such initiatives will not be repeated.

TAKE TIME TO REFLECT...

Here are some questions to reflect on as you focus on Presence. Think about how you might answer these today and how, through using the tips in this chapter, you might achieve a better result in the future.

When have you exhibited extraordinary courage? How were you able to move forward in spite of your fears? How can you leverage this approach to your benefit in future situations?

Where do you derive your self-confidence? How do you maintain it over time? How does it come across to others? What can you do to enhance the impact your confidence has on others?

Where are your fears constraining you? How have you been negatively affected by your lack of confidence and courage? What are you willing to do differently to overcome your anxieties? How will it translate into a stronger impact on others?

Where have you taken on a position of leadership or exhibited leadership characteristics without a formal title to do so? What positive impact were you able to bring to the situation? What did you learn from this experience that you can apply to other situations?

You can't lead a cavalry charge
if you think you look funny on a horse.

John Peers
American businessman and president of Logical Machine

25

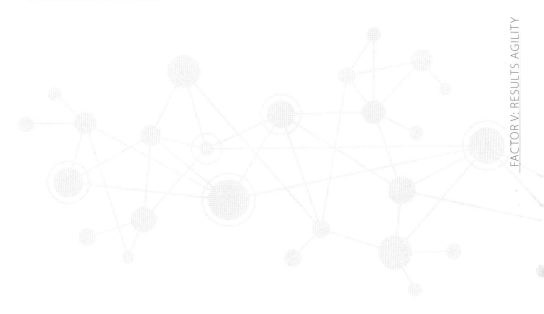

Inspires
Others

Inspiring others creates a positive shift in momentum. When your team should be feeling dispirited, they feel energized and uplifted instead. A master of momentum knows the right lever to pull at the right time with the right amount of force to get the desired results. While there are many tools available for motivating others, they must be applied with a surgeon's skill. Miscalculate, and energy can start flowing in the opposite direction. Successfully inspiring others requires a keen understanding of the situation and who you are dealing with combined with an intuitive sense of what needs to happen to change the dynamic in the right direction. Get the momentum started and it can begin to take on a life of its own. Suddenly you are getting pulled along rather than needing to tug. You have now turned the power of one into the power of many.

If your actions inspire others to dream more, learn more, do more and become more, you are a leader.

John Q. Adams
6th President of the United States

SKILLED

Taps into what motivates others
Creates a common purpose/shared mind-set
Raises others' confidence to tackle challenges
Reinforces teamwork and strong effort
Promotes high levels of energy and excitement

LESS SKILLED

Lacks commitment to goals and objectives

Expects others to be self-motivated

Overlooks hard work or accomplishments

Saps morale and enthusiasm

Focuses more on own performance

OVERUSE OF SKILL

Overinflates others' confidence

Raises energy and excitement to unsustainable levels

Overpraises; doesn't give enough constructive feedback

Focuses on inspiring at the expense of providing clear direction

SOME POSSIBLE CAUSES OF LOWER SKILL

Causes help explain "why" a person may have trouble in this dimension. When seeking to increase skill, it's helpful to consider how these might play out in certain situations. And remember that all of these can be addressed if you are motivated to do so.

Limited insight into others

Lacks caring or compassion

Self-centered

Lacks appreciation for others

Negative attitude

Overly critical

Poor communicator

Low energy

Out of touch

Unmotivated

Lacks commitment to goals

Expects others to be motivated the same way

DEVELOPMENTAL DIFFICULTY

When compared with other dimensions of Learning Agility, this dimension is **harder** to develop.

26

⭐ Does It Best

Sometimes efforts to inspire are carefully planned and targeted. Other times, inspiration can come about in very unexpected and unintentional ways. Take the example of Christopher Reeve. The inspiring impact of Reeve's portrayal of Superman was far exceeded by the qualities and actions he demonstrated when faced with real-life crises. When Reeve was paralyzed, it first shook the confidence and belief of many who viewed him as the indestructible Man of Steel. But the courage and commitment he demonstrated as he strived to recover from his injuries and advocate for treatment and cures for paralysis left no doubt as to his true strength. Christopher Reeve continues to serve as a symbol of motivation and hope for individuals with paralysis and for scientists seeking a cure.[22]

TIPS TO INCREASE SKILL IN INSPIRES OTHERS

Difficulty generating excitement?
Learn to engage hearts and minds.

ESTABLISH COMMON CAUSE
Nothing galvanizes people like a shared purpose, which is what holds any group together. Get everyone involved in sharing a common vision. Don't leave out the quiet or the reluctant. Repeatedly sell the logic of pulling together, listen, ask questions, invite suggestions to reach the outcome. Leave how things are to be done as open as possible. Specified sequences can be demotivating, even boring. People work harder under conditions of choice. Encourage experimentation.

LEARN TO READ PEOPLE'S MOTIVATION SIGNALS
What do they do first? What do they emphasize in their speech? What do they display emotion around? What values play out for them? Gathering person-specific insight in these areas unlocks the window into how to best motivate and inspire others.

- First things. Does this person go to others first, hole up and study, complain, discuss feelings, or take action? These are the basic orientations of people that reveal what's important to them. Use these to motivate.

- Speech content. People might focus on details, concepts, feelings, or other people in their speech. This can tell you again how to appeal to them by mirroring their speech emphasis. Although most of us naturally adjust—we talk details with detail-oriented people—chances are good that in problem relationships, you're not finding the common ground. She talks detail and you talk people, for example.

- Emotion. You need to know what people's hot buttons are because one mistake can get you labeled as insensitive with some people. The only cure here is to see what turns up the volume on their feelings.

- Values. Apply the same thinking to the values of others. Do they talk about money, recognition, integrity, efficiency in their normal work conversation?

WORK ON YOUR VISUAL SIDE

Learn storyboarding, a pictorial technique of representing a problem or process. Use mind mapping, a wonderfully branching way to plan, examine ideas, and simply think differently. Get some scenario training, then implement it with your team to come up with likely futures. Use flowcharting software packages. Close your eyes and see what the outcome would look like. Come up with an image or symbol that embodies the vision. People are much more likely to get excited by stories, symbols, and images than a white paper explaining the plan.

RESOURCES TO LEARN MORE

Harvard Business School Press. (2005). *Motivating people for improved performance.* Boston, MA: Author.

Kouzes, J. M., & Posner, B. Z. (2003). *Encouraging the heart: A leader's guide to rewarding and recognizing others.* San Francisco, CA: Jossey-Bass.

26

Carrying too much of the burden?
Tap into the power of teams.

KNOW THE BUILDING BLOCKS OF GREAT TEAMS
Here are five characteristics of high-performance teams:

1. They have a shared mind-set.

2. They trust one another—cover for each other, pitch in, are candid, deal with issues directly.

3. They have the talent collectively to do the job.

4. They operate efficiently, doing the small things well—running meetings, assigning work, dealing with conflict.

5. Most central to their excellence, they focus outside the team on customers and results. They do not focus much internally on atmosphere and happiness. Inward focus is a characteristic of low-performing teams who tend to delude themselves about their performance and focus on harmony.

SHIFT THE FOCUS FROM "ME" TO "WE"
Resistance to the idea of a team is best overcome by focusing on common goals, priorities and problems, selling the logic of pulling together repeatedly, listening patiently to people's concerns, protecting people's feelings but also reinforcing the perspective of why the team is needed, inviting suggestions to reach the outcome, and showing patience toward the unconverted. Maintain a light touch—a little well-timed humor goes a long way toward keeping spirits up in the face of significant challenges.

INSPIRE THE TEAM
Follow the basic rules of inspiring team members as outlined in classic books like *People Skills* by Robert Bolton or *Thriving on Chaos* by Tom Peters. Tell people what they do is important; say thanks; offer help and ask for it; provide autonomy in how people do their work; provide a variety of tasks; "surprise" people with enriching, challenging assignments; show an interest in their work; adopt a learning attitude toward mistakes; celebrate successes; have visible accepted measures of achievement, and so on. Each team member is different, so good team managers deal with each person uniquely while being fair to all.

If you find yourself creating a frenzy in others only to have inspiration slide away, ask yourself, "Do I believe what I am saying to others?" If you don't, neither will they—at least not for long. Make an effort to dial back your efforts at inspiring others so that they are actually aligned with your true convictions.

RESOURCES TO LEARN MORE

Capretta, C. C., Eichinger, R. W., Lombardo, M. M., & Swisher, V. V. (2009). *FYI™ for teams* (2nd ed.). Minneapolis, MN: Lominger International: A Korn/Ferry Company.

Wooden, J., & Jamison, S. (2005). *Wooden on leadership: How to create a winning organization.* New York, NY: McGraw Hill.

Efforts hard to sustain?
Learn to motivate for the long haul.

USE STRETCH GOALS TO MOTIVATE

Most people are motivated by reasonable goals. They like to measure themselves against a standard. They like to see who can run the fastest, score the most, and work the best. They like goals to be realistic but stretching. Research shows that people try hardest when they have somewhere between 1/2 and a 2/3 chance of success and some control over how they go about it. People are even more motivated when they participate in setting the goals. Set just-out-of-reach challenges and tasks that will be first time for people—their first negotiation, their first solo presentation, etc. Provide feedback and coaching along the way.

BUILD CONFIDENCE

Developing direct reports and others is dead last in skill level among the 67 competencies of the Leadership Architect® and has been since we started collecting these data. To develop people, you have to follow the essential rules of development. They take a bit of time. Development is not simply sending someone to a course:

- Start with a portrait of the person's strengths and weaknesses. They can't grow if they are misinformed about themselves.

- Provide ongoing feedback from multiple sources.

- Give them progressively stretching tasks that are first-time and different for them. Research shows that at least 70% of reported development occurs through challenging assignments that demand skill development. People don't grow from doing more of the same.

- Encourage them to think of themselves as learners, not just accomplishers. What are they learning that is new or different? What skills have grown in the last year? What have they learned that they can use in other situations?

26

· Use coursework, books, development partners, and mentoring to reinforce learning.

Because quality development is so rarely provided, the time you invest in developing your team not only increases skill, but serves as a boost to motivation and engagement.

COACH AND DELEGATE

People aren't motivated when you give them the answer or, even worse, step in to do things for them. They become dependent and unfulfilled. Alternatively, teaching and skill building, even when it involves a challenging learning experience, is motivating and empowering. To boost learning, always explain your thinking. Work out loud with them on a task. What do you see as important? How do you know? What questions are you asking? What steps are you following? Resist temptation to blurt out the answer. Let them reach their own conclusion. Don't intervene before minor mistakes happen. Treat them as learning opportunities.

RESOURCES TO LEARN MORE

Sirota, D., Mischkind, L. A., & Meltzer, M. I. (2005). *The enthusiastic employee: How companies profit by giving workers what they want.* Upper Saddle River, NJ: Prentice Hall.

Steinfeld, J. (2012, April 18). 5 Things great mentors do. *Inc.com*

ASSIGNMENTS TO PRACTICE SKILL

Get buy-in and commitment from others on an important change initiative. Seize the opportunity to establish a shared vision and utilize different messages and symbols to spark and sustain motivation.

Assemble a team of diverse people to accomplish a difficult task where you can't go it alone and others are integral to success. Tap into their motivation triggers to help them be successful.

Turn around a low-performing, disengaged team. This will require you to play multiple roles (coach, teacher, guide, mentor, etc.) while rebuilding their motivation and performance.

TAKE TIME TO REFLECT...

Here are some questions to reflect on as you focus on Inspiring Others. Think about how you might answer these today and how, through using the tips in this chapter, you might achieve a better result in the future.

What can you do to better inspire followership? Where could someone feel herded or driven rather than inspired and led? What will you do to understand your team members' perceptions?

Do you know what inspires and motivates those around you? What can you do to better understand their needs and wants? How can you best leverage this understanding to influence and motivate?

When have you been surprised at a decreasing or fleeting motivation in others? What contributed to this? What could you have done to sustain a heightened level of motivation over time?

How much time do you spend on creating messages? When have you left a conversation or message only to think, "I could have said that better"? What can you do to sharpen the clarity of what you say to others? How can you better use messages to motivate and inspire others?

Pretend that every single person you meet has a sign around his or her neck that says, 'Make Me Feel Important.' Not only will you succeed in sales, you will succeed in life.

Mary Kay Ash
American entrepreneur

26

Delivers
Against the Odds

Sometimes it seems like there's just no way to accomplish your goal. The problem is extraordinary in scope. The resources are few or none. The time is short. The obstacles appear insurmountable. Yet, in the end, you triumph. That's the difference when you have the ability to deliver against the odds. You find a way despite all the difficulty, struggle, and apparent hopelessness to persevere and accomplish your goal. Delivering against the odds requires some occasional luck, but the ability to get consistent results under difficult circumstances is no accident. It's an amalgam of focus, determination, resilience, and a willingness to take risks. Put it all together, and you get an impressive ability to make things happen. Developing the ability to deliver against the odds won't guarantee you the outcomes you're seeking, but you will see your success rate increase. And when you do fall short of your goal, you will still embrace the experience because of the lessons you can glean from it—turning what on the surface may seem like a failure into a launchpad to future success.

The only way to discover the limits of the possible
is to go beyond them into the impossible.

Arthur C. Clarke
British author, inventor, and futurist

SKILLED
Is a go-to person in tough situations
Maintains a clear and steady focus on meeting goals, despite obstacles
Perseveres in the face of difficulties
Is resilient when encountering setbacks and failures
Succeeds where others have fallen short

FACTOR V: RESULTS AGILITY

LESS SKILLED
Prefers familiar situations with a high probability of success

Shirks difficult responsibilities

Gives up easily when faced with challenges

Often comes up short of meeting objectives

Makes excuses; avoids accountability

OVERUSE OF SKILL
Takes unnecessary risks

Quickly loses interest if things aren't challenging enough

Makes things harder than they need to be

Pushes too long, too far, too hard; continues to invest effort and resources in a lost cause

Engages in questionable tactics or compromises values to make things happen

SOME POSSIBLE CAUSES OF LOWER SKILL
Causes help explain "why" a person may have trouble in this dimension. When seeking to increase skill, it's helpful to consider how these might play out in certain situations. And remember that all of these can be addressed if you are motivated to do so.

Low risk orientation

Prefers certainty and familiarity

Non-competitive

More concerned with the journey than the destination

Lacks resilience

Easily upset

Low focus

Pessimistic

Lacks confidence in self/others

Overreliant on others

Low standards for success

DEVELOPMENTAL DIFFICULTY
When compared with other dimensions of Learning Agility, this dimension is **easier** to develop.

27

⭐ Does It Best

In the annals of adventuring, perhaps no tale stands out as incredible as Ernest Shackleton's ill-fated expedition to Antarctica in 1914. After the team's ship became trapped and eventually crushed in sea ice, the goal switched from successfully crossing the Antarctic continent to one of simple survival. Over the course of 14 months, Shackleton and his team traversed over 1,000 miles of ice and open ocean with no more than a few row boats and limited provisions to finally reach civilization. In the end, not a single life was lost. Reflecting on his harrowing journey, Shackleton remarked, "Superhuman effort isn't worth a damn unless it achieves results."[23]

TIPS TO INCREASE SKILL IN DELIVERS AGAINST THE ODDS

Struggling under pressure?
Build your defenses.

USE MENTAL REHEARSAL FOR TOUGH SITUATIONS

Learn to recognize the clues that you're about to fall back on an unproductive behavior and be ready with a fresh strategy that you have decided in advance. If you know, for example, that a solution isn't working and you're likely to be questioned about it, be ready to engage others and get the benefit of their thinking instead of pointing fingers and making excuses.

STUDY YOUR DAILY TRANSITION POINTS

It's all in a day's work—going from a tense meeting to a celebration for a notable accomplishment. The mental and emotional whiplash that results from these jarring transitions can be unnerving and lead to slipups. To begin getting the upper hand on your transitions, study them closely. For a week, monitor your gear-shifting behavior at work and at home. What transitions give you the most trouble? The least? Why? Practice gear-shifting transitions. On the way between activities, think about the transition you're making and the frame of mind required to make it. Reflect on how smoothly you made each transition and the resulting impact on your behavior.

RECOGNIZE YOUR FRUSTRATION AND ANXIETY TRIGGERS

Research shows that initial anxious responses last 45–60 seconds. They are marked by your characteristic emotional response. Learn to recognize your triggers (raising your volume, drumming your fingers, shifting in your chair, etc.). Once you have figured out your triggers, ask why these are a problem. Is it ego? Extra work? People you dislike or think are lazy? For each grouping,

27

figure out what would be a more mature response. If it's too late, count to 10 or ask a clarifying question. Stall until the initial burst of glucose and adrenaline subsides.

RESOURCES TO LEARN MORE

Berent, J., & Lemley, A. (2010). *Work makes me nervous: Overcome anxiety and build the confidence to succeed.* Hoboken, NJ: John Wiley & Sons, Inc.

Burton, K. (2010). *Live life, love work.* West Sussex, England: Capstone Publishing Ltd.

Hesitant response?
Dive in.

START NOW

You don't go back a second time until forced to by deadlines? Less motivated when your first attempt falls flat or meets resistance? Don't get back to people when you said you would? You might not produce results consistently. Some of your work will be marginal because you only had time for one or two attempts before the project was due. Start earlier. Reduce the time between attempts. Always start 10% of each attempt immediately after it is apparent it will be needed so you can better gauge what it is going to take to finish it. Always assume it will take more time than you think it's going to take.

BALANCE THOUGHT WITH ACTION

Break out of your examine-it-to-death mode and just do it. Sometimes you hold back acting because you don't have all the information. Some like to be close to 100% sure before they act. Anyone with 100% of the data can make good decisions. The real test is who can act the soonest with a reasonable amount, but not all, of the data. Some studies suggest successful general managers are about 65% correct. If you learn to make smaller decisions more quickly, you can change course along the way to the correct decision. You may examine things to death because you are a chronic worrier who focuses on the downsides of action. Write down your worries, and for each one, write down the upside (a pro for each con). Once you consider both sides of the issue, you should be more willing to take action. Virtually any conceivable action has a downside, but it has an upside as well. Act, get feedback on the results, refine, and act again.

LEARN TO TAKE CALCULATED RISKS

Won't take a risk? Sometimes producing results involves pushing the envelope, taking chances, and trying bold, new initiatives. Doing those things leads to more misfires and mistakes but also better results. Treat any mistakes or failures as chances to learn. Nothing ventured, nothing gained.

Up your risk comfort. Start small so you can recover more quickly. See how creative and innovative you can be. Satisfy yourself; people will always say it should have been done differently. Listen to them but be skeptical. Conduct a postmortem immediately after finishing. This will indicate to all that you're open to continuous improvement, whether the result was stellar or not.

Are you an "adrenaline junkie"? Pushing the envelope for the rush that comes with narrowly averting disaster? Stop to consider the potential consequences for yourself as well as others. Don't curb your desire or willingness to take risks, just be mindful of the risk you are taking and what might happen as a result.

RESOURCES TO LEARN MORE

Branson, R. (2010, November 1). The art of calculated risk. *Entrepreneur*.

Corporate Executive Board Staff. (2011, December 20). Preventing "analysis paralysis." *Bloomberg BusinessWeek*.

Confidence shaken?
Reframe and regroup.

DEVELOP A PHILOSOPHICAL STANCE TOWARD FAILURE/CRITICISM

After all, most innovations fail, most proposals fail, most efforts to lead change fail. Anything worth doing takes repeated effort. Anything could always have been done better. Research says that successful general managers have made more mistakes in their careers than the people they were promoted over. They got promoted because they had the guts to lead, not because they were always right. Other studies suggest really good general managers are right about 65% of the time. Put errors, mistakes, and failures on your menu. Everyone has to have some spinach for a balanced diet.

PUT ADVERSE REACTIONS IN PERSPECTIVE

Don't persevere because you prefer to avoid conflict? Hesitate in the face of resistance and adverse reaction? Conflict slows you down? Shakes your confidence in your decision? Do you backpedal? Give in too soon? Try to make everyone happy? When your initiative hits resistance, keep it on the problem and the objectives. Depersonalize. If attacked, return to what you're trying to accomplish and invite people's criticisms and ideas. Listen. Correct if justified. Stick to your point. Push ahead again. Resistance is natural. Some of the time it's legitimate; most of the time it's just human nature. People push back until they understand. They are just protecting territory.

TRY SOMETHING DIFFERENT

If you have trouble going back the second or third time to get something done, then switch approaches. Sometimes people get stuck in a repeating groove that's not working. Do something different next time. If you visited the office of someone you have difficulties with, invite him/her to your office next time. Think about multiple ways to get the same outcome. For example, to push a decision through, you could meet with stakeholders first, go to a single key stakeholder, study and present the problem to a group, call a problem-solving session, or call in an outside expert. Be prepared to do them all when obstacles arise.

RESOURCES TO LEARN MORE

Bregman, P. (2009, April 28). How to counter resistance to change. *Harvard Business Review*.

Hess, E. D. (2012, June 20). Creating an innovation culture: Accepting failure is necessary. *Forbes*.

ASSIGNMENTS TO PRACTICE SKILL

Stretch yourself and others to deliver a tough project on time and on budget. This will require you to demonstrate resilience, vigilance, and composure to make it through to completion.

Take responsibility for something beyond what you think you can do. Be willing to risk failure in order to achieve greatness and embrace the whole experience as an opportunity to learn and grow.

Take over a failing project. Engage in rapid experimenting and real-time damage control while keeping the team on task toward its goal.

TAKE TIME TO REFLECT...

Here are some questions to reflect on as you focus on Delivers Against the Odds. Think about how you might answer these today and how, through using the tips in this chapter, you might achieve a better result in the future.

Where have you allowed the process, obstacles, or constraints to interfere with achieving a goal? How might you approach situations differently if you focus only on the end in mind? What will you do differently to focus your actions more toward seeing the solution?

Where have you seen your strengths rise to meet a challenging situation? How might they have gone untested in less adverse situations? What types of situations will you seek out to further hone your talents?

When have you struggled the most to achieve success? What contributed to the challenge? Why did you struggle? What did you learn about yourself as a result? What do you (or will you) do differently as a result of this learning? What will you change?

Where can you attribute some of your professional success to an earlier failure? What learnings did you derive from the failure that caused changes that led to more effective outcomes?

....

Because a thing seems difficult for you,
do not think it impossible for anyone to accomplish.

Marcus Aurelius
Roman emperor and philosopher (121 CE – 180 CE)

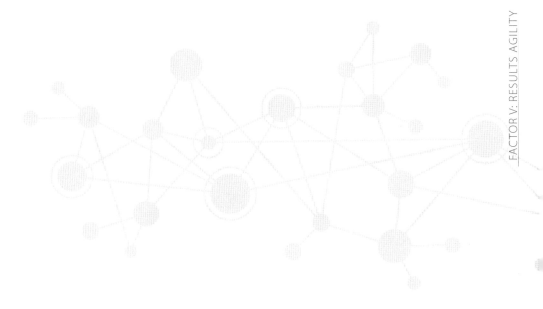

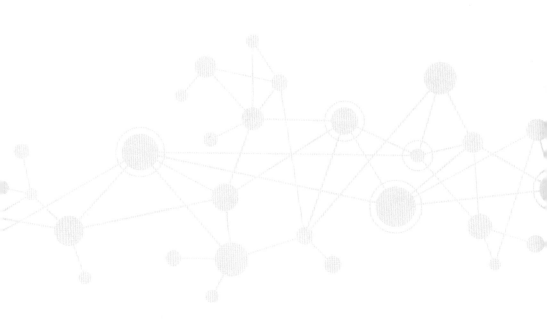

Acknowledgments

A number of people contributed to the creation of this book and deserve a great deal of thanks and appreciation.

Thanks to Heather Barnfield, Guangrong Dai, Jon Feil, Dana Landis, and King Yii (Lulu) Tang for their thoughtful review and insights throughout the writing process.

A special thanks to Jon Feil for providing such a variety of useful additions for the "Resources to Learn More" sections in each chapter.

Appreciation goes out to Zoe Hruby, Nicole Lambrou, Steve Marshall, and Kim Ruyle for their valuable input into content and formatting enhancements.

The content publishing team of Lesley Kurke, Doug Lodermeier, Paul Montei, and Bonnie Parks did a top-notch job of proofing, editing, design, layout, and production.

Finally, thanks to the Learning Agility Architect™ core team of Kirk DiFrancesco, Molly Hedlund, Lisa Niesen, Valerie Petit, La Tasha Reed, and Allison Rufsvold for their efforts in making this book a reality.

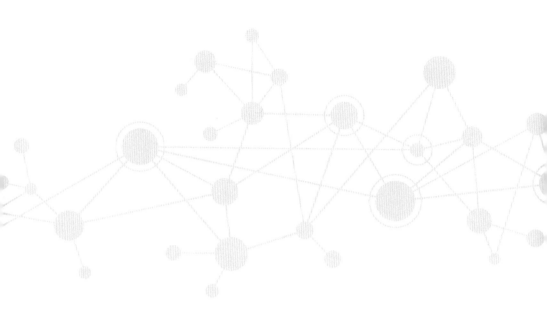

Development Plan

The following pages provide you with a Development Plan template where you can record your development need and action plan.

PERMISSION TO COPY DEVELOPMENT PLAN: This confirms that Lominger International: A Korn/Ferry Company is granting you the right to make copies of My Development Need on pages 252–255 of *FYI™ for Learning Agility* 2nd Edition. Such copies are for the internal use of your organization only. All copies must retain the copyright notice located on the bottom of each page.

My Development Need: *(Sample)*

Dimension 20: Experimenter

Factor IV: Change Agility

LEARNER NAME:...

TO BE COMPLETED BY:...

MY "BEFORE" DESCRIPTION (LESS SKILLED)	SOME POSSIBLE CAUSES OF LOWER SKILL
Like to have everything just so.	*Don't like taking risks.*
Hold changes up to impossibly mature standards.	*Fear failure and making mistakes.*
	Perfectionist.

WHAT I LEARNED ABOUT THIS DIMENSION OF LEARNING AGILITY

I will not be able to innovate unless I am willing to experiment and fail. If I can decrease the risk involved and increase the number of tries, I will be able to learn a lot from early experiments.

QUOTES THAT INSPIRE ME

"A life spent making mistakes is not only more honorable, but more useful than a life spent doing nothing." – George Bernard Shaw

MY ACTION PLAN (TIPS AND ASSIGNMENTS)	MY "AFTER" DESCRIPTION (SKILLED)
Turn the monumental into the manageable—start small, get feedback, make adjustments, and build up to bigger risks. *Be philosophical about failure/ criticism. When we make mistakes ask, "What can we learn from this?"* *(Assignment) Relaunch an existing product or service that's not doing well. Experimenting with unvetted ideas will be welcomed since it's obvious the "usual suspect" solutions haven't worked.*	*View failures as opportunities for learning.* *See mistakes as a necessary part of the innovation process.*

DEV. PLAN

RESOURCES I WILL USE TO LEARN MORE

How to start the big project you've been putting off. Harvard Business Review.

My Development Need:

....

....

LEARNER NAME:..

TO BE COMPLETED BY:..

MY "BEFORE" DESCRIPTION (LESS SKILLED)	SOME POSSIBLE CAUSES OF LOWER SKILL

WHAT I LEARNED ABOUT THIS DIMENSION OF LEARNING AGILITY

QUOTES THAT INSPIRE ME

MY ACTION PLAN (TIPS AND ASSIGNMENTS)	MY "AFTER" DESCRIPTION (SKILLED)

DEV. PLAN

RESOURCES I WILL USE TO LEARN MORE

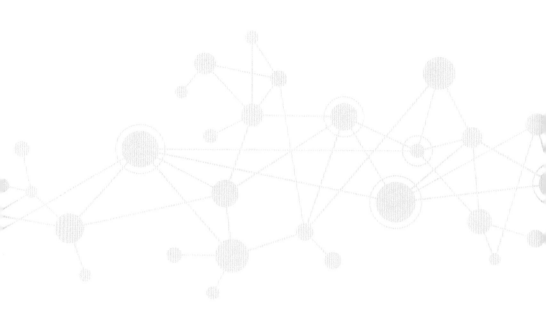

Appendix

Resources to Learn More – Web Addresses

SELF-AWARENESS

Personal Learner

Beh, E. (2012). Powerful guidelines on effectively writing a personal development plan. *Self-Improvement Mentor*. Retrieved from http://www.self-improvement-mentor.com/writing-a-personal-development-plan.html

Buxton, B. (2011). Always be a beginner. Business Innovation Factory. Retrieved from http://www.businessinnovationfactory.com/iss/stories/always-be-a-beginner

Grant-Halvorson, H. (2011, February 1). Why letting yourself make mistakes means making fewer of them. *Psychology Today*. Retrieved from http://www.psychologytoday.com/blog/the-science-success/201102/why-letting-yourself-make-mistakes-means-making-fewer-them

Kopp, W. (2011, January 20). Advice for social entrepreneurs [Video file]. Stanford Technology Ventures Program. Retrieved from http://www.youtube.com/watch?v=TUAS1iY1f7s

Feedback Oriented

Bell, M. (2012). Why you need to ask for feedback from others. *Business Know-How*. Retrieved from http://www.businessknowhow.com/growth/askfeedback.htm

Donnelly, T. (2010, August 10). How to get feedback from employees. *Inc.com*. Retrieved from http://www.inc.com/guides/2010/08/how-to-get-feedback-from-employees.html

Heathfield, S. M. (2012). Receive feedback with grace and dignity. *About.com*. Retrieved from http://humanresources.about.com/cs/communication/ht/receivefeedback.htm

Houlihan, M. (2012, September 21). Oops, my bad! 5 Ways your business can improve by admitting to mistakes. *Entrepreneur*. Retrieved from http://www.entrepreneur.com/article/224491

Reflective

Addison, M., & Pavelich, K. (2012, March 20). Embracing our perfect imperfect selves. [Video file]. TEDxThunderBay. Retrieved from http://www.youtube. com/watch?v=AgcA_q9RRlk

Goodreads. (2012). Popular thought provoking books. *Goodreads.com*. Retrieved from http://www.goodreads.com/shelf/show/thought-provoking

Paul, R., & Elder, L. (2001). Critical thinking in everyday life: 9 Strategies. The Foundation for Critical Thinking. Retrieved from http://www.criticalthinking. org/pages/critical-thinking-in-everyday-life-9-strategies/512

Stamos-Kovacs, J. (2012). Blissing out: 10 Relaxation techniques to reduce stress on-the-spot. *WebMD*. Retrieved from http://www.webmd.com/balance/ guide/blissing-out-10-relaxation-techniques-reduce-stress-spot

Emotion Management

Bregman, P. (2010, June 10). The no-drama rule of management. *Harvard Business Review*. Retrieved from http://blogs.hbr.org/bregman/2010/06/i-lay-back-in-the.html

Cain, M. (2011, October 13). Don't take this personally, but you take things too personally. *Forbes*. Retrieved from http://www.forbes.com/sites/ glassheel/2011/10/13/dont-take-this-personally-but-you-take-things-too-personally/

Graham, C. (2010, April 2). Be well at work, learn to pause…erase that blur! *Corporate Wellness Magazine*. Retrieved from http://www. corporatewellnessmagazine.com/article/be-well-at-work.html

Mayo Clinic Staff. (2012, July 21). Exercise and stress: Get moving to manage stress. Mayo Clinic. Retrieved from http://www.mayoclinic.com/health/exercise-and-stress/SR00036

Muzio, E. (2011, January 26). The ladder of inference creates bad judgment [Video file]. Retrieved from http://www.youtube.com/watch?v=K9nFhs5W8o8

Self-Knowledge

Ingram, D. (2012). What are the benefits of 360 degree feedback? *Chron.com*. Retrieved from http://smallbusiness.chron.com/benefits-360-degree-feedback-1929.html

Reddy, K. (2012, February 27). Now, don't get defensive, but… *Financial Post*. Retrieved from http://business.financialpost.com/2012/02/27/now-dont-get-defensive-but/

Vajda, P. (2007, December 13). Asking co-workers for feedback. *Helium*. Retrieved from http://www.helium.com/items/745204-asking-co-workers-for-feedback

Winfrey, O. (2000, December). Oprah talks to Maya Angelou [Interview]. *O, The Oprah Magazine*. Retrieved from http://www.oprah.com/omagazine/Oprah-Interviews-Maya-Angelou/3#ixzz20Qf2lQfi

MENTAL AGILITY

Inquisitive

Blakely, D. (2011, March 14). Fostering innovation [Video file]. Stanford Graduate School of Business. Retrieved from http://www.youtube.com/watch?v=xS01QlLMvzI

Reilly, J. M. (2012, April 18). Embracing failure on the path to success. *Entrepreneur*. Retrieved from http://www.entrepreneur.com/article/223366

Rubin, G. (2009, November 12). *The happiness of doing something new: The audiobook version*. The Happiness Project. Retrieved from http://happiness-project.com/happiness_project/2009/11/the-happiness-of-doing-something-new-the-audiobook-version/

Broad Scanner

Biography Channel. Retrieved from www.biography.com

Fast Company. Retrieved from www.fastcompany.com

Connector

Day, P. (2009, June 23). Mind of a millionaire. BBC series.

[Video file 1 of 6]. Retrieved from http://www.youtube.com/watch?v=kzQXdArhgSU

[Video file 2 of 6]. Retrieved from http://www.youtube.com/watch?v=c4-0FzH_D-k

[Video file 3 of 6]. Retrieved from http://www.youtube.com/watch?v=bs632llpZ44

[Video file 4 of 6]. Retrieved from http://www.youtube.com/watch?v=Bcf10RmCTzw

[Video file 5 of 6]. Retrieved from http://www.youtube.com/watch?v=AsQCLLrHlgI

[Video file 6 of 6]. Retrieved from http://www.youtube.com/watch?v=zXNHwEyRPiI

Shaughnessy, H. (2011, June 24). The new work manifesto: Be unconventional. *Forbes*. Retrieved from http://www.forbes.com/sites/haydnshaughnessy/2011/06/24/the-new-work-manifesto-be-unconventional/

Essence

Grohol, J. M. (2012). 15 Common cognitive distortions. *Psych Central*. Retrieved from http://psychcentral.com/lib/2009/15-common-cognitive-distortions/

Hodnett, E. (2010). Determine the root cause: 5 Whys. Six Sigma. Retrieved from http://www.isixsigma.com/tools-templates/cause-effect/determine-root-cause-5-whys/

Complexity

Friedman, S. (2008, April 11). A more holistic approach to problem solving. *Harvard Business Review*. Retrieved from http://blogs.hbr.org/friedman/2008/04/a-more-holistic-approach-to-pr.html

McLeod, L. E. (2011, March 17). How to solve really big problems. *HuffingtonPost.com*. Retrieved from http://www.huffingtonpost.com/lisa-earle-mcleod/how-to-solve-really-big-p_b_833793.html

Manages Uncertainty

Curiosity.com. (2011). Is it OK to fail? [Video file]. Retrieved from http://curiosity.discovery.com/question/failure-okay

Girard, K. (2009, May 4). Three tools to manage uncertainty. CBS News. Retrieved from http://www.cbsnews.com/8301-505125_162-51295091/three-tools-to-manage-uncertainty/

Johri, V. (2010, March 9). Leaders today have to be comfortable with ambiguity. *Business Standard*. Retrieved from http://www.business-standard.com/india/news/leaders-today-have-to-be-comfortableambiguity/21/29/387898/

Robbins, M. (2010, September 13). 4 Simple ways to let go of control. *Huffington Post*. Retrieved from http://www.huffingtonpost.com/mike-robbins/let-go-of-control_b_710620.html

PEOPLE AGILITY

Open Minded

Cutts, M. (2011, July). Try something new for 30 days [Video file]. Retrieved from www.ted.com/talks/matt_cutts_try_something_new_for_30_days.html

Johnson, K. (2012, May 31). Get to know people [Video file]. Retrieved from http://www.youtube.com/watch?v=T157AI3iTog

Lickerman, A. (2010, April 1). Trying new things. *Psychology Today.* Retrieved from www.psychologytoday.com/blog/happiness-in-world/201004/trying-new-things

LinkedIn Discussion Forums. (2011, August 25.) How to stay objective when facing conflict between team members? Linkedin.com. Retrieved from http://www.linkedin.com/answers/management/labor-relations/MGM_LBR/882498-7413879

People Smart

Johnson, K. (2012, May 31). Get to know people [Video file]. Retrieved from http://www.youtube.com/watch?v=T157AI3iTog

Situational Flexibility

AttitudeTVChannel. (2010, May 9). Sam Glenn's airplane story [Video file]. Retrieved from http://www.youtube.com/watch?v=6qdbPdl1fKA

Agile Communicator

Brown, P. B. (2006, September 2). Listen up. Know your audience. *New York Times.* Retrieved from http://www.nytimes.com/2006/09/02/business/02offline.html

Gallo, C. (2009, March 24). Presentation lessons you didn't learn in B-school. *Bloomberg Businessweek.* Retrieved from http://www.businessweek.com/smallbiz/content/mar2009/sb20090324_710581.htm

Simon, S. (2009, June 12). How to tell a story. National Public Radio Weekend Edition. Retrieved from http://www.youtube.com/watch?v=tiX_WNdJu6w

Conflict Manager

Winfrey, O. (2001, April). Oprah talks to Nelson Mandela [Interview]. *O, The Oprah Magazine.* Retrieved from http://www.oprah.com/world/Oprah-Interviews-Nelson-Mandela/7#ixzz20QwtP6Ai

Helps Others Succeed

Basheer, T. (2008). 10 Ways to be a good mentor. Blue Sky Coaching. Retrieved from www.blueskycoaching.com.au/pdf/v4i10_mentor.pdf

Garner, E. (2012). *Delegation and empowerment: Giving people the chance to excel.* [eBook version]. Retrieved from http://bookboon.com/en/business-ebooks/management-ebooks/delegation-and-empowerment

Pink, D. (2009, August 25). The puzzle of motivation [Video file]. Retrieved from www.ted.com/talks/lang/en/dan_pink_on_motivation.html

Spiro, J. (2010, April 16). How to delegate properly. *Inc.com*. Retrieved from www.inc.com/guides/2010/04/how-to-delegate-properly.html

CHANGE AGILITY

Continuous Improver

Best, M. (2012, May 14). Get the corporate antibodies on your side. *Harvard Business Review*. Retrieved from http://blogs.hbr.org/cs/2012/05/get_the_corporate_antibodies_o.html

Bloomberg Businessweek. (2008, December 4). Managing stress can improve company performance. *Bloomberg Businessweek*. Retrieved from http://www.businessweek.com/stories/2008-12-04/managing-stress-can-improve-company-performance

Branson, R. (2010, November 1). The art of calculated risk. *Entrepreneur*. Retrieved from http://www.entrepreneur.com/article/217479

Crom, M. (2012, February 3). Answer tough questions with honesty, explanation. *USA Today*. Retrieved from http://tinyurl.com/bsp9gc8

Cutts, M. (2011, July). Try something new for 30 days [Video file]. Retrieved from www.ted.com/talks/matt_cutts_try_something_new_for_30_days.html

Visioning

Hansen, M. (2010, January 21). IDEO CEO Tim Brown: T-Shaped stars: The backbone of IDEO's collaborative culture. *Chief Executive.net*. Retrieved from http://chiefexecutive.net/ideo-ceo-tim-brown-t-shaped-stars-the-backbone-of-ideoae%E2%84%A2s-collaborative-culture

Watkins, M. (2007, April 20). How to think strategically. *Harvard Business Review*. Retrieved from http://blogs.hbr.org/watkins/2007/04/how_to_think_strategically_1.html

Experimenter

Bregman, P. (2012, February 9). How to start the big project you've been putting off. *Harvard Business Review*. Retrieved from http://blogs.hbr.org/bregman/2012/02/how-to-start-the-big-project-y.html

Girard, L. (2012). Five creativity exercises to find your passion. *Entrepreneur*. Retrieved from http://www.entrepreneur.com/article/219709

Pychyl, T. A. (2008, March 26). Just get started. *Psychology Today*. Retrieved from http://www.psychologytoday.com/blog/dont-delay/200803/just-get-started

Innovation Manager

Basulto, D. (2010, April 25). Before you innovate, understand the business model of your industry. Future Lab. Retrieved from http://www.futurelab.net/blogs/marketing-strategy-innovation/2010/04/you_innovate_understand_busine.html

Hess, E. D. (2012, June 20). Creating an innovation culture: Accepting failure is necessary. *Forbes*. Retrieved from www.forbes.com/sites/darden/2012/06/20/creating-an-innovation-culture-accepting-failure-is-necessary/

McKinney, P. (2012, February 17). Beyond the obvious: Killer questions that spark game-changing innovation [Video file]. Retrieved from http://www.youtube.com/watch?v=ITAxR8oQUu0

Comfort Leading Change

Adams, S. (2012, June 18). Eight ways goofing off can make you more productive. *Forbes*. Retrieved from http://www.forbes.com/sites/susanadams/2012/06/18/eight-ways-goofing-off-can-make-you-more-productive/

Russell, J. E. A. (2010, September 13). Career coach: A key element of successfully managing change. *The Washington Post*. Retrieved from http://www.washingtonpost.com/wp-dyn/content/article/2010/09/10/AR2010091006532.html

RESULTS AGILITY

Drive

Geller, L. (2012, July 25). Getting out of your comfort zone. *Forbes*. Retrieved from http://www.forbes.com/sites/loisgeller/2012/07/25/getting-out-of-your-comfort-zone/

Masie, E. (2007, August 24). Three cheers for stretch assignments. *Chief Learning Officer*. Retrieved from http://clomedia.com/articles/view/1906

Pink, D. (2009, August 25). The puzzle of motivation [Video file]. Retrieved from www.ted.com/talks/lang/en/dan_pink_on_motivation.html

Resourcefulness

Baldoni, J. (2010, January 13). The importance of resourcefulness. *Harvard Business Review*. Retrieved from blogs.hbr.org/baldoni/2010/01/leaders_can_learn_to_make_do_a.html

Laufenberg, D. (2010, December). How to learn? From mistakes [Video file]. Retrieved from www.ted.com/talks/diana_laufenberg_3_ways_to_teach.html

Nauert, R. (2012, October 3). Work is rewarding when personal traits match job. *Psych Central*. Retrieved from psychcentral.com/news/2012/10/03/work-is-rewarding-when-personal-traits-match-job/45475.html

Presence

Andersen, E. (2012, July 23). 3 Simple ways to discover your passion. *Forbes*. Retrieved from http://tinyurl.com/95ez7ny

Fenson, S. (2000, March 1). Want to be more effective? Learn to listen. *Inc.com*. Retrieved from www.inc.com/articles/2000/03/17491.html

Stevenson, W. H., III. (2011, February). Cutting out filler words. Toastmasters. Retrieved from http://tinyurl.com/8m2vb8r

Inspires Others

Steinfeld, J. (2012, April 18). 5 Things great mentors do. *Inc.com*. Retrieved from http://www.inc.com/jay-steinfeld/5-ways-to-be-a-better-mentor.html

Delivers Against the Odds

Branson, R. (2010, November 1). The art of calculated risk. *Entrepreneur*. Retrieved from http://www.entrepreneur.com/article/217479

Bregman, P. (2009, April 28). How to counter resistance to change. *Harvard Business Review*. Retrieved from blogs.hbr.org/bregman/2009/04/how-to-counter-resistance-to-c.html

Corporate Executive Board Staff. (2011, December 20). Preventing "analysis paralysis." *Bloomberg BusinessWeek*. Retrieved from http://www.businessweek.com/management/preventing-analysis-paralysis-12202011.html

Hess, E. D. (2012, June 20). Creating an innovation culture: Accepting failure is necessary. *Forbes*. Retrieved from www.forbes.com/sites/darden/2012/06/20/creating-an-innovation-culture-accepting-failure-is-necessary/

Notes

SELF-AWARENESS

Personal Learner

1. Raina Kumra. (2011, June 23). Retrieved from http://wearenytech.com/169-raina-kumra-senior-new-media-advisor-u-s-department-of-state

    Safian, R. (2012. February). The secrets of generation flux. *Fast Company, (162)*, 60–97 [Special Issue].

Feedback Oriented

2. Angelou, M. (2004). *The collected autobiographies of Maya Angelou*. New York, NY: Random House.

Reflective

3. Center for Creative Leadership, & Teachers College of Columbia University. (2013). The 5 practices to increased learning agility [Webinar]. Available at http://www.ccl.org/leadership/community/fiveWebinar.aspx?sp_rid=913a5837-0761-4be2-802d-df52f77046f5&sp_mid=39739906

Self-Knowledge

4. Church, A. H. (1997). Managerial self-awareness in high-performing individuals in organizations. *Journal of Applied Psychology, (82)*2, 281–292.

5. Orr, J. E., Swisher, V. V., Tang, K. Y., & De Meuse, K. P. (2010). *Illuminating blind spots and hidden strengths* [White Paper]. Minneapolis, MN: Korn/Ferry Institute.

MENTAL AGILITY

Inquisitive

6. Isaacson, W. (2007). *Einstein: His life and universe*. New York, NY: Simon & Schuster.

Connector

7. Gill, C. (2012). Dyslexia can be "route to riches." *Mail Online*. Retrieved from http://www.dailymail.co.uk/news/article-198603/Dyslexia-route-riches.html#ixzz26BpNNxlu

8. Pink, D. (2005). *A whole new mind: Why right brainers will rule the future*. New York, NY: Penguin Group.

Essence

9. Gladwell, M. (2009). *What the dog saw and other adventures.* New York, NY: Back Bay Books.

Complexity

10. Orr, J. E. (2012). *Becoming an agile leader: A guide to learning from your experiences.* Minneapolis, MN: Lominger International: A Korn Ferry Company.

PEOPLE AGILITY

Open Minded

11. Goodwin, D. K. (2005). *Team of rivals: The political genius of Abraham Lincoln.* New York, NY: Simon & Schuster.

People Smart

12. Matlin, M. W. (2009). *Cognition* (7th ed.). New York, NY: John Wiley and Sons, Inc.

Situational Flexibility

13. U2, & McCormick, N. (2009). *U2 by U2.* New York, NY: HarperCollins Publishers.

Agile Communicator

14. 1992 Presidential Debate. (Uploaded 2007, June 5). Clinton's debate moment [Video file]. Retrieved from http://www.youtube.com/watch?v=ta_SFvgbrlY

Conflict Manager

15. The Elders. (2013). Retrieved from http://www.theelders.org/

Helps Others Succeed

16. Renwick, P. A., & Lawler, E. E. (1978, May). What you really want from your job. *Psychology Today,* 53–65.

CHANGE AGILITY

Continuous Improver

17. Safian, R. (2012, January 9). Generation flux: Beth Comstock. *Fast Company.* Retrieved from http://www.fastcompany.com/1806752/generation-flux-beth-comstock

Visioning

18. de Vries Hoogerwerff, M. (2007, November 7). Interview with Lee Kuan Yew [Video file]. Retrieved from http://www.youtube.com/watch?v=B3YFl-dY9Qg

Experimenter

19. Walker, T. (2012, September 20). Sir James Dyson's innovation awards inspire some of the smartest and oddest new inventions. *The Independent*. Retrieved from: http://www.independent.co.uk/life-style/gadgets-and-tech/features/sir-james-dysons-innovation-awards-inspire-some-of-the-smartest-and-oddest-new-inventions-8157368.html

Innovation Manager

20. Grossman, L., Thompson, M., Kluger, J., Park, A., Walsh, B., Suddath, C., Dodds, E., Webley, K., Rawlings, N., Sun, F., Brock-Abraham, C. & Carbone, N. (2011, November 28). The 50 best inventions. *Time Magazine*. Retrieved from http://www.time.com/time/magazine/article/0,9171,2099708-1,00.html

Comfort Leading Change

21. Kim, W., & Mauborgne, R. (2003). Tipping point leadership. *Harvard Business Review, 81*(4), 60–69.

RESULTS AGILITY

Inspires Others

22. Christopher & Dana Reeve Foundation. Retrieved from (http://www.christopherreeve.org/site/c.ddJFKRNoFiG/b.4048063/k.C5D5/Christopher_Reeve_Spinal_Cord_Injury_and_Paralysis_Foundation.htm)

Delivers Against the Odds

23. Lansing, A. (2007). *Endurance: Shackleton's incredible voyage*. New York, NY: Basic Books. (Original work published in 1959.)

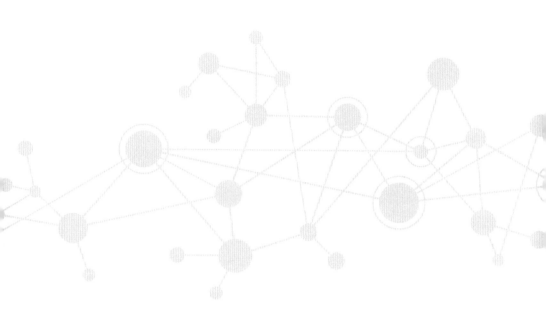

Additional Resources

Research has clearly shown that Learning Agility is a primary component and key differentiator of potential for leadership roles. By understanding and leveraging Learning Agility in your organization, you can better distinguish between current performance and future potential and create a more targeted, differentiated development strategy for current and future leaders. The assessment and development tools here can help you integrate Learning Agility into your organization's strategic talent management initiatives.

ASSESSMENT TOOLS

viaEDGE™ easily and efficiently gauges the Learning Agility of large numbers of individuals, with the ease of an online self-administered assessment. viaEDGE™ helps organizations assess internal talent for placement and development of high potentials and can aid in external candidate hiring. *Available in multiple languages.*

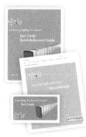

The Choices™ multi-rater assessment has been used for years by organizations to identify, validate, and select those who are the most learning agile. Choices™ scores have been significantly related to independent measures or ratings of potential, consistent performance, and staying out of trouble. Other formats available and branded as part of the Learning Agility Architect™ suite are the Sort Cards and a Quick Score Questionnaire. *Available in multiple languages.*

Selecting an Agile Leader: Find Future-Ready Talent Today and the Learning From Experience™ Interview Guide are designed to provide an in-depth assessment of Learning Agility through an interview process. *Selecting an Agile Leader* is a book that provides the context and benchmarks to improve interviewer rating accuracy. The Learning From Experience™ Interview Guide is an interview template that provides questions, prompts, and themes to listen for, and a rating scale to use during the interview. Both are designed to help organizations build future bench strength through interviewing and selecting the most learning agile internal and external candidates.

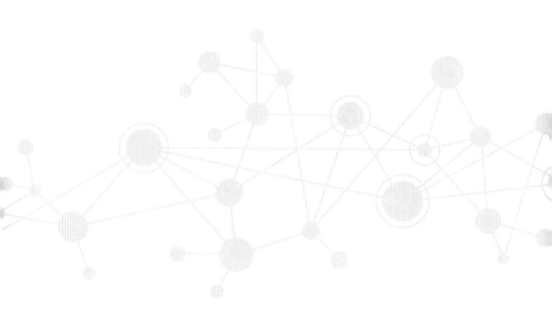

DEVELOPMENT TOOLS

Learning Agility can be developed. Here are some tools that can help you on your journey to explore and potentially build your Learning Agility.

Becoming an Agile Leader: Know What to Do…When You Don't Know What to Do explores the five key characteristics, or factors, of Learning Agility. Spotlighting well-known leaders from business and the world stage, *Becoming an Agile Leader* is filled with more than 70 practical development tips you can start using today to increase your own agility and help ensure success in those new, challenging assignments. So you will know what to do…when you don't know what to do.

With *Becoming an Agile Leader: A Guide to Learning From Your Experiences,* you can explore the formative experiences that shaped the learning agile leaders profiled in the book *Becoming an Agile Leader.* This practical guide lets you reflect on your own experiences, past and present, and includes a comprehensive listing of on- and off-the-job experiences that will help you plan for assignments that build Learning Agility.

The *Becoming an Agile Leader* Reflections App can help you achieve greater self-awareness through capturing on-the-spot insights and reflections. The *Becoming an Agile Leader* Reflections App provides inspiring, thought-provoking quotes related to the Learning Agility factors that help you easily reflect, document, and transfer lessons from your experiences.

FYI™ for Insight will help you understand 21 leadership characteristics for success and 5 characteristics that can derail your career. It will also make you aware of *why* you may be lacking skill or motivation in certain areas. This is critical because becoming self-aware can get you 50% of the way toward improving your performance.

Insight into strengths and weaknesses can help you get what you want from your career. The *FYI™ for Insight* Self-Awareness Assessment is a three-step process that takes just a few minutes. A personalized report gives you a self-awareness score and highlights your hidden strengths and blind spots.

More information on these resources can be found at http://www.lominger.com